A
Blind
Autobiography

By

Professor Derek Hull

Assisted by

Karen L. Hull

D1323674

The right of Derek Hull to be identified as the author of this
work has been asserted in accordance with Section 78
of the Copyright, Designs and Patents Act 1988

The book cover picture is copyright to Derek Hull

This book is published by
Grosvenor House Publishing Ltd
Link House
140 The Broadway, Tolworth, Surrey, KT6 7HT.
www.grosvenorhousepublishing.co.uk

A CIP record for this book
is available from the British Library

ISBN 978-1-78623-265-6

Thank you to everyone who has offered me help, love and support,
particularly my dear wife, Pauline.

And special thanks to my daughter, Karen.
Without her immense input this book would not have been achievable.

Royalties from the sales of this book will be donated
to various eye charities including:
The Macular Society, Royal National Institute for the Blind,
Wirral Society for the Blind and Partially Sighted.

Foreword

To walk in another man's shoes is a beguiling thought and a near impossible task. To read an autobiography allows a taste of the past, the present and indeed the possible future of the writer. Like all good stories, it begins with a fascinating life. My father's life has been rich in endless ways and I hope that the reader will find much to tease his interest as he strolls through each chapter, opening doors for a glimpse at the kaleidoscope of events that have shaped my father and the many people who have influenced his world.

This book, *A Blind Autobiography*, whilst scrupulously autobiographical, is not restricted by the constraints of a rigorous timeline. Its underlying theme; the difficulty of accepting and living with the onset of blindness and Age-related Macular Degeneration, meanders through more than four score years of episodes in the various stages of my father's life. It examines and reflects upon the impact of the increasing disability of sight impairment on a man, whose journey has taken him from a lower middle-class family through the corridors of physics, metallurgy and research, to the high tables of Cambridge University and beyond, and combines his immense interest in science with anecdotal narrative to paint the picture.

This is not, and was never meant to be a self-help book, but it is a valuable insight into the physical and psychological struggle he has faced when presented with the challenge of sight loss. It is certainly not a medical textbook but rather a gentle conversation that you would have with an old friend. It is informative yet reassuring, allowing the reader to gain gentle access to a knowledge and understanding of this increasingly common ailment. It examines progressive eye disease from a patients' point of view and extends a warm narrative to offer empathy, consolation and hope to a fellow sufferer.

Sadly, loss of sight is not uncommon, and my father's is not a solitary tale, but it is unique. Like so many health issues that afflict a vast proportion of people, living with sight loss is a shared experience. The ripples from the inevitable changes in lifestyle, roles and independence, radiate silently to eddy the waters of connected lives. In painting for you the colourful pictures of his past, he is describing and defining his life with sight in order to illuminate what is being lost, to hint at the frustration of a future depleted of colour, and to convey a compassion for everyone, sufferers and carers, friends and relatives, who find themselves within the encompassing circle of sight loss. This is a blind man's story and I leave the vision in the hands of the reader.

Karen Hull

Contents

Chapter 1

Opening Thoughts

Why does one write a book? Why does one write an auto-biography? There must be numerous reasons. Hopefully, by the end of this book, there will be a few answers to these rather abstract questions. It is far easier to describe the circumstances that triggered the idea of writing. I need to go back almost eighty-seven years to my birth in the Lancashire mill town of Blackburn in 1931 between the two Great Wars. Life doesn't owe me anything. Although my brother David and I were born into a relatively poor family, we were cared for and supported by loving parents. Despite the war years, we had a good education and were fortunate to go to good universities. Chance and good fortune followed us throughout our lives. With our wives, we have been blessed with loving children who have shared their lives with us and produced another generation of bright, loving and creative children: yet another generation is following. Many opportunities opened-up to David and me with challenging and exciting career paths, the fortuity to visit all parts of the world and to be involved in numerous assignments in university, government and industrial environments.

David was 361 days younger than me when he was born with a twin brother who died at birth. Under these circumstances, it is not surprising that in our early years we were very close. Perhaps I was the absent twin. In our spare time, particularly in school holidays, we did every-thing together. Not having many books in our home, we filled our time with 'projects' guided by numerous practically-oriented hobbies described in the family's ten-volume set of books of Arthur Mee's *Children's Encyclopaedia*. This way of using time has influenced most of my non-professional activities throughout my life. In many hobbies, David and I were aided and abetted by our mum who was skilled in all things related to handicrafts. One of our early projects was focused on butterflies and moths (Lepidoptera). For two or three years we spent most of our summer holidays scour-ing the fields and hills around our new home in Blackpool. We collected these beautiful insects and preserved them to display in spectacular arrays. Thus, it was, that filling time with engrossing projects became one of the main ways of having an absorbing and satisfying life. I don't think that either David or I had the right genes or inclinations to adopt a geekish-type of enthusiasm for any of our projects – life had other plans for our long-term futures and careers. However, I still have an inner need to fill my time with pro-jects without a burning desire to make them into lifetime commitments. Bear in mind I am referring to hobbies, not career. So, in later life, a high proportion of my time was spent with hobbies involving photography, marquetry, bird-watching, fell walking, art, enamelling, poetry and heathers as well as golf and crown green bowls.

I started going to the eye clinic at Arrowe Park Hospital, Wirral in May 2000, but it is only four and a half years since my eyesight started to deteriorate with AMD (Age-related Macular Degeneration) in such a way that my activities were affected. Eventually, I had to make the decision to stop driving both on roads and on golf courses. As most of my projects depend on very good eyesight these types of projects had to be abandoned. This resulted in the inevitable question, 'What can I do that is creative, challenging and good fun?'

I discussed this dilemma with my 61-year-old son Andrew. He lives in Sweden and we regularly have long conversations on topics as diverse as the origin of the universe and the prospects of a soft Brexit. Recently, I had a conversation in a call from Sweden a day or so after a session with my AMD consultant. After reviewing all the notes in a thick case folder and examining recent test results, the consultant confirmed my own feelings that my eyes had deteriorated significantly. It was decided that I should be registered as SPS (Severely Partially Sighted). In much of the literature about eyes, SPS is followed by the rather bleaker term of 'blind'. This confirmation of my eye situation sent some distress signals to my brain. What was I going to do? One approach might be to rely on listening solutions such as music, audiobooks and radio.

Andrew is fully aware of my need to get involved with projects. He has a mathematical PhD from Imperial College London. He responded to my dilemma with a rather provocative observation that Leonhard Euler, a brilliant pure mathematician of the 18th century, had produced some of the best of his mathematical work when he was totally blind and over sixty years old. The mind boggles. Strangely, though not a mathematician, I knew of some of Euler's work in the context of a relatively simple concept he produced about the instability of rigid elastic columns subjected to axial compression. Two hundred years later this analysis was used to analyse the behaviour of fibre reinforced composites. The work was one of the themes of a university textbook that I published with Cambridge University Press in 1981 – it is still in print.

In my professional career, I have written four books and with my research students and colleagues, I published about 240 scientific and technological papers. Is there something worth saying about blindness? How did Euler 'think' mathematics without sight? Andrew opined that Euler was probably surrounded by many intellectual colleagues who shared his mathematical enthusiasm and supported him in formulating and publishing his work. I think the term for this sort of assistance is amanuensis, but don't quote me! I felt my best option for a book that I could write relating to blindness, would be based on my own experiences since I had no knowledge of professional work on ophthalmology, optometry, medical conditions and treatments, eye care etc. Andrew was persuasive and told me I had a family team who would give me lots of support, albeit not trained in eye issues: a daughter who is a hospital consultant specialising in autism, a daughter who is a dentist and implant surgeon, a daughter who has a first-class degree in mathematical physics and has been employed in a well-known computer company, a daughter who manages a large primary school, and a wife who looks after me and, in her spare time, achieved two honours degrees via The Open University. She is an amazing woman who at the tender age of 86 years is still the permanent church organist.

My title *A Blind Autobiography* is intended to emphasize that the book is 'experientially' based. In contrast, most scientific literature is based on an extensive review of previous work, as recorded in the recognised literature, coupled with sophisticated experimental work and theoretical analysis.

There is little scope, in an experientially-based work, for the inclusion of vast contributions from Google.

As numerous authors have testified, writing can be a tough pursuit. With very limited sight the prospects of writing a book are doubly challenging. In the past, when my sight was good, I produced initially a succession of rough notes on the subject matter, before producing a draft copy for typing. This was subjected to revisions before submission to the editor and publisher.

With little sight, I anticipated that it would be difficult for me to follow this sequence—and so it proved. In a later chapter, I explain the methods I used to transfer words created in my brain into a text that could be accessed by normal word processing and into hard copy. Throughout the writing process, I had a concern that my deteriorating sight might highjack my attempts to complete the work.

All the stories in this book relate to my own experiences and all have some connection with blindness. I sense a lack of balance in the choice of chapters because only six of my 86 years have been troubled by blindness. In some respect, this is inevitable. My hope and intention has been to address themes that have a broad aspect both to blindness and to individual and personal concerns about being blind.

For example, the sixth chapter of the book really relates to the importance of volunteering which is manifest in the activities of the Macular Society through the massive support it gives to the blind community by its encouragement and recruitment of volunteers. But volunteering depends on strictly personal decisions and can be seen to be rooted in one's life story: childhood, family, career and a host of very personal experiences.

The theme in the chapter about golfing and walking may be more obscure. The stories remind me of a life full of fun and excitement as a result of joining with friends in many different circumstances. I suppose that even struggling with blindness, the blind man enjoys the challenges of walking in tough conditions. There is an extra special experience when the sight of some can aid those who are struggling with the absence of sight.

You are invited to search this book to seek other themes and to share these ideas with others.

Chapter 2

The Day War Broke Out

"The day war broke out", on Sunday 3 September 1939, my younger brother David and I watched our Dad open his 'closed-Sunday' shop. He crossed the busy road and disappeared into a ramshackle shed in the grounds of the Red Lion pub. When he returned home he told his wife and two young sons that he had volunteered and signed up as an air raid warden. For the five years of the war, he oversaw a team of wardens. They met in a brick shelter protected by twelve inches of reinforced concrete. Our family lived above the shop in a suburb of the famous Lancashire town of Blackpool. Compared to the Blitz bombing of the port of Liverpool, only 28 miles away, we had a quiet war. The community kept a diligent watch to protect people and property. Children carried gas masks to school.

The opening phrase of the above paragraph was the inspiration of a comedian Rob Wilton, who was born in Everton. He was the source of much laughter and hearty chuckles on stage and radio as the author of many famous monologues. Through his stories, we are invited to picture a middle-aged couple slouched beside a small coal fire. The wife berates her husband about the war effort. She challenges and teases him. The weary man tells the story,

"The day war broke out, my missus said to me: 'It's up to you... You've got to stop it!' I said, 'Stop what?' She said, 'The war!'" Was she hinting that her man should join the Dad's Army?

My dad knew about war. He was only seventeen years old when World War I started. I suppose he went back to a job in the cotton industry after the war, re-joining his family living in Blackburn, Lancashire. My younger brother David and I are very lucky that Dad met Nellie Hayes, probably at Park Road Congregational Church where they were both Sunday School teachers. By the time they were married, Dad had opened a small greengrocers shop at 157, Bolton Road in Blackburn and it was here that they were living when I arrived. The family left for Blackpool before my memory has any recall. The shop was taken over by Dad's brother Walter, and I have some memories of the place from returning to visit him later. It was a tiny corner shop on the main road out of Blackburn (pronounced Blakbun) to Darwen (pronounced Darren) and Bolton (pronounced Bowtun – if you say them quickly). On the opposite side of the cobbled road was a large cotton mill with its massive gates and chimneys. A few yards along the road was the canal (the cut) with a towpath. On match days, crowds of men, many in clogs, streamed past the shop along Bolton Road on their way to see Blackburn Rovers. W.S. Lowry has provided many vivid images of the mills of Lancashire – it was just like that. We lived behind the shop. There were only a small living room and a kitchen downstairs. Outside, across the tiny yard, was the toilet. I can't remember any-thing about the upstairs rooms, which were approached by narrow stairs directly from the living room. There was no bathroom, so bathing the baby, and everybody else pre-sumably, was with the help of a galvanised tub in the kitchen. This gives colourful meaning to the saying: "I'll scrub your back, if you'll scrub mine". My only memory of Grandad Hull, who died when I was nine, was on a visit to Uncle Walter in Bolton Road. Grandad, by then living with Uncle Walter, was sitting in a rocking chair by the side of the coal fire. I will never know if he knew that I existed but there are photographs to say that he did.

Yes, my dad knew about war. Mum and Dad were married on June 5, 1930 at Park Road Congregational Church in Blackburn. They were a good-looking couple. The marriage certificate informs that Dad was in 'retail fish and fruit' which is a posh way of saying a greengrocer who sells fish. By this time, Dad had abandoned the cotton industry because world recession had resulted in massive redundancies in the industry and the depression was biting hard in Blackburn. After leaving school at the age of thirteen or fourteen, he had become an apprentice in the industry following in his father's footsteps; he trained at night school in the skills of draughtsman and technical work related directly to the design and operation of cotton making machinery. I saw some of his drawings: they always impressed me. As I said, he was only seventeen when the Germans invaded France at the start of World War I in 1914. He was an early volunteer and joined the Royal Corps of Signals rising to the rank of corporal. In those days, the messages were sent down wires using Morse code and so it is not surprising that I remember a Morse code tapper in our home and that I learnt Morse code early in my life. Dad was unable to talk much about his wartime experiences; they were so horrible, as many television documentaries have shown us in recent years. Occasionally he opened up, when David and I were in our teens, to recall the terrifying effects of his war in France, of constant artillery bombardment, the water filled trenches, the arrival of opposition tanks across the fields so that survival depended on how quickly a soldier could dig a trench so that the tanks went over him, the Christmas Day experiences of fraternising with the enemy and, for me, the most frightening experience of having, under orders and the threat of being shot for desertion, to climb out of the trenches under a hail of bullets and charge towards the enemy a few hundred yards away. He was injured and yet still went back to fight. His brother Jesse was not so lucky: he didn't return. Is it any wonder that our generation still pauses at the eleventh hour of the eleventh day of the eleventh month of each year to remind ourselves of the horror of war and the exact time that the Armistice was signed to end World War I in 1918? On a school visit to the fields of France, one of my grandsons visited the Thiepval Memorial where Jesse is remembered in stone. There was no body to recover for burial.

We moved to Blackpool when I was four years old. At the time, Blackpool was a relatively prosperous seaside resort. Mum and Dad started a greengrocers shop at 1 Lowmore Road in Greenlands, a small community on the outskirts of Blackpool and it was here that I grew up, from where I went to school and from where I got married. As yet, no plaque has been posted on any of the relevant buildings! David and I went to Bispham Endowed Church of England Primary School in the village of Bispham at the northern end of the Blackpool promenade. I can't remember a thing I was taught at Bispham Primary School, but I could take you on an imaginary journey through all the classrooms and introduce you to all the teachers. There is one thing I still think about. The headmaster walked up and down the aisles in the classroom with a cane in his hand trying to persuade us that coal stocks in the world would be exhausted within forty years. I worried about keeping warm.

The day World War II ended I was trapped in bed with scarlet fever. The best I could do was listen to the celebrations in the street. World War II ended with the unconditional surrender of the Axis powers. On Tuesday 8 May 1945, the Allies accepted Germany's surrender, about a week after Adolf Hitler had committed suicide. VE Day – Victory in Europe Day, celebrated the end of the Second World War on 8 May, 1945.

I was now at Baines Grammar School, founded in 1717, and was making good but not spectacular progress. My admission to the school was 'touch and go'. I didn't achieve a sufficient standard in what is now called 'the 11-plus test or SAT's' to allow me to attend the local grammar school. Somehow my dad heard about Baines Grammar School which was nestled in the countryside a few miles from Blackpool. Did he hear about it from a customer at the shop? Baines had a Prep school and a facility for admission to the main school through an entrance examination. I was entered into this examination and was successful. I give my dad all the credit for this and I am convinced that his initiative was founded on the principle that he was determined that his children would be encouraged to have a far better opportunity than he had had. For me, the joy of this story is the memories I have of returning home on the Saturday morning after the exam and telling my Dad, who was standing behind the counter in the shop, what I had done. He beamed with pride about the essay I had written on the theme 'A Windy Day'. For the first three years of my days at Baines, I had to take an envelope containing three guineas and walk to the front of the class to present it to the form teacher to pay the fees. My dad was relieved of the expense at the end of three years when the government introduced a new Education Act.

Baines was a good school for me. Many of the male staff had been recruited to the armed forces and had been replaced by relatively young female teachers. A few seasoned male staff were left behind, and I give top marks to Mr 'King' Peel for teaching me mathematics – now long forgotten.

I have included this story because it fills me with a sense of gratitude to my mum and dad. It amazes me that Dad, immersed in war and the depression of the 1930s was able to support his family in all sorts of ways. Brother David and I remain deeply indebted to our parents.

My success with the essay in the entrance exam was not repeated in my English performance at Baines School. I cringe at the memories. I will mention only two essays that still haunt me. The first of these had the seemingly simplistic title of 'My Favourite Room'. I hated writing stories and was thoroughly bad at writing. I thought teachers were over-enthusiastic at creating abstract topics to drain the brains of their students. I have changed my mind a bit over the years, however, that is another story. The chore of trying to write essays often extended for hours for me. It was a laboured effort, finding the right words, expressing something worthwhile and most importantly, at least so it seemed at the time, preventing me from spending any time playing with my friends. Eventually, I appealed to my dad for help with this essay. 'He' got ten out of ten from the teacher, who might have recognised plagiarism! The second essay has teased my brain for many years and now seems rather poignant as a discussion point since it particularly relates to this blind autobiography. It can also prove quite a good topic for a dinner party when all other conversation has stuttered to an awkward lull. It was the question:

'Which of the senses is most precious?'. Then, I voted for sight and made an absolute mess of the essay writing blindly (if you will excuse the pun) on the relative merits, if there can be any, of becoming blind compared with becoming deaf. Nowadays, my vote is cast for the common conclusion that the feeling of isolation experienced by those who are hard of hearing puts hearing above sight in the 'precious' list. Perhaps, as a young lad, I had experienced some of the wonderful sights of my small world but had yet to hear the beauty of the music of Beethoven!

As a teenager, I had the same problems that all teenagers have when deciding a plan for the rest of my life. It is always a nagging question which often takes priority over the appreciation of the more fragile, esoteric world. I still have memories of two incidents which affected my thinking at that time.

One, in particular, tells some revealing points. Around the age of fifteen, I wrote a proposal for my future in some detail which involved me setting up a company that would have a chain of greengrocers – a natural development from my dad's one-man corner shop. It was a funky written up proposal and one evening after the shop closed and my dad had put his feet up by the fire I presented it to him and retired to bed. I got his reply the next morning which was a resounding: "No chance! You will stick at grammar school to get as far as you can!" I didn't resist.

There was another voice at that time when King Peel reported in my annual school report, commenting on my mathematical skills with: "Derek has a quick grasp of the subject but fails to truly follow up". I wouldn't resist this analysis as an epithet on my life and it could be used for many aspects of my forty years as an academic – but don't press me for details.

As I moved into my late teenage years there is evidence of enthusiasm and application. As we shall see this wasn't always successful. My ability and skills responded by winning local athletics competitions and school sports particularly in sprinting. I was joint captain of Baines athletics team and we won a major Inter Grammar Schools annual games. Elsewhere, I spent some years as a Cadet in the school's Air Training Corps (ATC) Squadron becoming Flight Sergeant and being selected at a national level to represent the United Kingdom on a major tour of Canada.

There were bigger challenges at an academic level. My results at Higher School Certificate level, now called A-Level, were very respectable but in those days admission to university was dominated by the admission of men and women who had served in the armed forces; they had priority. The first time around, I was not successful. I was hoping to read physics or metallurgy. I was particularly hoping to read physics with the idea of teaching physics to blind children, however, my interviews were a bit like my essays. After another year in the sixth form, I tried again concentrating on metallurgy. I got more refusals despite an excellent in scholarship physics. My Achilles' heel was a simple pass on School Certificate English which was not regarded to be sufficient for matriculation. My luck finally held when the University of Wales introduced a special admission clause in which, for two or three years, mainly for the benefit of ex-service people, a pass in English was acceptable. Hurrah for Wales and Cardiff, and for Professor W.R.D. Jones who was totally delighted when I got a First-Class Honours degree in 1953 – the same year in which Queen Elizabeth became Queen of England, Edmund Hilary and Tenzin climbed Everest, Blackpool Football Club won the FA Cup, and Pauline Scott married Derek Hull.

Chapter 3

The Academic Years

My next forty years are best described as academic; however this needs some explaining. It is dominated by flexibility, the opportunity to choose, the emphasis on personal ability for pursuing a field of study and learning for oneself, the will to say no or reject financial reward and the glory road, coupled with the pressure to be the best one can be and contribute to the progress of studying intellectual subjects wherever they lead. It is a massive challenge but a great privilege to have the opportunity. Progress in the disciplines is so dependent on the ability to choose and to be subject to the changes and chances of the fleeting world. I drew a really, wonderful straw.

My choice of metallurgy was determined, in part by the write-ups in university prospectuses that suggested that the courses would be attractive to students with equal strengths in physics, chemistry and mathematics. I seemed to meet this requirement without being particularly good at any of these important scientific disciplines. I later learnt from schoolboy 'chat' that metallurgy was 'the second oldest profession'. Before arriving at University, I wrote to the Head of Department and ask him if there was anything I could usefully do in the long summer vacation to prepare me for my newly discovered subject of metallurgy. He was a wise man and suggested that I find a vacation job in a factory working in this field. My hometown of Blackpool was not at the heart of the industrial North. I was lucky to be taken on at a steel casting works at the fishing port of Fleetwood. Here, large iron components were produced to replace damaged parts of seagoing trawlers. Huge furnaces were used to produce cast iron which was poured into moulds made from heavily compacted sand. There was plenty of scope for accidents and the workforce was a tough crowd of friendly men, with a language of their own, who introduced me to the great university of life, and the seamier parts of English literature not normally taught to sixth formers of a grammar school.

University College Cardiff and a sister college in Swansea were constituent colleges of the University of Wales. The metallurgy department at Cardiff was the first university in the UK to award metallurgy degrees. They provided a massive source of learning for the whole of the industry of South Wales, dominated by the mining of coal, and the ferrous and non-ferrous metal industry. I was in the right place to study metallurgy and I thoroughly enjoyed my studies and the people who welcomed me. I was attracted most to the physical side of metallurgy which as it emerged was developing into a powerful discipline. At the core, there is an understanding of the relationship between the performance and properties of metals and the underlying internal structure which, in simple terms, is the arrangement of the atoms. Engineers needed new and advanced materials including metals, ceramics and plastics to make stronger and more durable structures: for ships, aeroplanes, cars, washing machines, etc. More powerful optical and electron microscopes were needed to explore the internal structures, and advanced mathematical studies were needed to interpret and understand the real and complex relationships between these structures and their properties.

As I recall my holiday experiences and university, I could digress and tell you about the magic of understanding some of the crucial issues about my own personal research that I did, the outcome and understanding of which was crucially dependent on the ability to see very clearly and accurately. This is a background story to the whole of my research life, yet some of the work that I did is still as real and thoroughly exciting as it was during those hours sitting at the bench beside a microscope in my old university. However, it also occurs to me that I do not have the time and ability to tell you about the rest of my research career in anything like the detail I have offered so far. So, I will not attempt to fill in the detail of the next thirty-five years except for a few highlights to tell you how they shaped my life.

I cannot resist telling you about martensite. This was the major theme in my final year project at university. As students, we were given the choice of several different projects. My choice was influenced by the lecturer who was to supervise my work and guide it, and by the underlying challenges that it offered.

In those days, martensite was the name given to a select kind of steel that is exceptionally hard, and it is widely used today. The name derives from a German scientist called Adolf Martens who first identified it around 1890. This material has a special composition of mostly iron, carbon and small amounts of other elements which are heated up to about 900°C and then quenched into cold water. The temperature is well below the melting point of the steel and in the process of the quenching, the movement of the atoms in the steel creates a very special kind of structure or microstructure. Quenching in water prevents the atoms in the steel from moving into the same position as they would have if the steel was cooled slowly. My supervisor introduced me to a special kind of martensitic process which had been discovered in some brass and bronze alloys, and the work which had been published in scientific papers in the USA. We needed to know more and wanted to see it happening in real time. In some brass, the transformation occurs at below 0°C. When I searched the literature, an essential discipline for a researcher, I found several abstracts of work by a Russian professor, published in Russian ten years earlier. Professor Kudjumov with his students had found a way of watching the transformation in real time. I wanted to repeat his experiments and study the martensitic transformation. Much of the project involved setting up a special microscope and designing a system for cooling a metal specimen and following the transformations or changes which occurred as it was cooled and heated. There was a special difficulty in avoiding the condensation of water from the surrounding atmosphere on to the surface that resulted in the formation of brilliant ice crystals since these obscured the changes in the metal sample. Needless to say, this experiment would be impossible for students without keen eyesight.

The really exciting part of this work was watching and recording the change in the patterns which sprung rapidly to view as the transformations occur and the martensite formed – a process that happened very rapidly and was reversed when the cooling was reversed. The patterns were mesmerizing, exotic and photogenic. From a scientific

approach, the biggest challenge was to measure and interpret the arrangement of the complex pattern of straight
lines in terms of the orientation of the underlying distribution of the atoms within the crystals of the metal specimen.
My work was found acceptable and, after three years of
metallurgical study, I graduated in 1953.

The year 1956 was a big year for our family and for my
career. I was nearly persuaded to accept an offer to do a
PhD degree at Oxford but eventually decided to continue
my adventures with martensite at Cardiff for another
three years. I didn't have to decide about signing on for
National Service during my PhD studies. So, having married
before commencing my PhD, Pauline and I settled in a
utility bungalow in Llandaff, near Cardiff. Following three
exciting years of research, Pauline offered to type my
PhD thesis. Computers had not been invented yet; it was
painstakingly laborious work on a typewriter. There was
one difficulty, our first baby was due at the end of April and
so there was a big race between completing the thesis
and the arrival of the baby. The thesis won, but shortly
afterwards we joyously received the real prize. Andrew
was born on 24 April and was christened Andrew Martin.
I wonder why?

Soon I had to make the biggest decision of my academic career. The options were National Service, an offer
of employment with a major international nuclear energy
company or a position as a Scientific Officer at the Atomic
Energy Research Establishment (AERE) at Harwell in
Berkshire. Both nuclear appointments were seeking to
develop the peaceful potential of nuclear energy which was
regarded as work of national importance. My lovely Cardiff
professor had strong views, but I put the AERE opportunity

at the top of my list of interviews. More luck than good management.

My visit to AERE for an interview was exciting in many ways. I travelled from Cardiff to Didcot, a few miles from Harwell, by train and was advised by railway staff to use the last carriage. When I got off the train at Didcot, I stood alone on the platform and watched the train as it disappeared into the far distance, leaving only the last solitary, stationary carriage. I heaved a thankful sigh of relief. Outside the station, I was greeted by a uniformed chauffeur with a large car and taken to the Metallurgy Division building, where I was to be interviewed by the Head and Deputy Heads of the Division. They turned out to be two of the most distinguished metallurgists in the country. The Head of the division, Dr Monty Finniston (later Sir Monty) spent the best part of half an hour extolling the importance of manual dexterity and was very proud of his own handwriting, which I had difficulty reading. He was keen to emphasize the importance of experimental scientists having the skills necessary for complex experimental techniques. Dr A.H. Cottrell (later Sir Alan) had joined Harwell one or two years earlier and quizzed me at length about my ability to write reports and scientific papers. I think the fact that I had recently achieved first prize for a paper on defining the martensitic transformation, which had been published, helped me a lot.

I joined Harwell in September 1956 and got even more good news when Director Monty informed me that he had developed a scheme with Sir Francis Simon, Head of the Clarendon Laboratory, the world famous low-temperature physics laboratory in the University of Oxford, for the secondment of one of his scientific officers to spend 50% of their time in Oxford and 50% in Harwell, and that he wanted me to do it. So, I was then fortunate enough to do my research in Harwell and Oxford – wonders never cease! And, there was an added bonus, for at the metallurgy department at Oxford there was a senior academic who was a world specialist on a theoretical understanding of martensitic transformations.

I spent over three years researching many topics directly related to the use of materials in the atomic energy industry. They were exciting years since this was a new industry which was involved in developing completely new applications for materials under demanding conditions which had not been experienced before. As the technology developed and the industry matured, the time came for me to move on to new challenges. An opportunity arose at the University of Liverpool through personal contacts and I joined the Metallurgy Department as a Lecturer in 1960. The incumbent, charismatic Head of Department (HOD) soon moved on for appointments in the States, and I became a professor and the new head. One of my key objectives was to widen the discipline and approaches which had developed in physical metallurgy to other classes of materials such as glasses, plastics or polymers, ceramics and eventually composite materials. I was able to hire high-quality new staff and I also adjusted my own subject interests to encourage these changes. We were fortunate to be able to recruit new research students and post-doctoral staff and attract substantial funds for our research from government and industrial sources.

The next thirty-five years have been full of massive opportunities and do not add too much to my academic story. As an academic in a university system, I accepted responsibilities such as Dean of Engineering and Pro-Vice Chancellor, as well as an endless stream of committee duties such as the car parking committee! As a researcher, I published with my students over two hundred papers and two graduate textbooks. I interacted with industrial research laboratories involved in problems common to my own interests. For a year, I was a National Science Foundation Fellow at the University of Delaware, USA. I served on many government bodies and through my research contacts, I visited countries including Australia, South Africa, Japan, Finland, Sweden, Switzerland, France, Germany and Chile.

My days in Liverpool stopped in 1984 when I was invited to be the Goldsmiths Professor and Head of Department of Metallurgy and Materials Science at The University of Cambridge. I had eight years of excitement with far too many stories to tell. My duties included being a Professorial Fellow of Magdalene College and in those eight years, I was elected a Fellow of the Royal Academy and a Fellow of the Royal Society. For added benefit, we lived close to the Botanic Gardens and we were within a short cycle distance of my university department, my college, the main railway station, the river Cam and the United Reformed Church. However, the North Sea coast was unfortunately about forty miles away.

Chapter 4

Writing Books

Good question, why write a book? This is a question like why climb Everest, or why try to sail to the North Pole through the vast melting ice? A popular answer is 'because it is there'. This response hides all sorts of intangible issues and is open to challenges by those who have not experienced the excitement of big adventures. A cynic has a problem with the idea of writing for blind people who cannot see to read a book. Part of my answer is given in chapter 1. I have an inbuilt need to do something challenging and interesting: a 'project'. Unfortunately, with very poor eyesight most of the activities I was familiar with are no longer possible. So, perhaps I could write a book even though it may be impossible.

There are many approaches to writing books. There is always a challenge. I have published four books in over fifty years. The first was called *An Introduction to Dislocations* and was published in 1956. After leaving Harwell, I lectured at the University of Liverpool and, as part of my duties, developed a final year honours lecture course on dislocations which are atomic-scale defects in crystalline solids. The book has been in print for fifty-six years and there have been four new editions with extensive rewriting to include changes in this important scientific subject. After the second edition, I was joined by another scientist with an extensive knowledge of dislocations. The book has been published in five other languages including Russian and Japanese.

The inspiration for the book must be credited to the Head of Department in Liverpool who had developed close contacts with the distinguished publisher Robert Maxwell, who had created a large scientific publishing house called Pergamon Press which specialised in sciences, engineering and medical books. Those with good memories will recall that Maxwell (MP and MC) was the owner and chief editor of the *Daily Mirror* before he died in a tragic sailing event. He was larger than life and a very creative man. The book was aimed at undergraduate and postgraduate students in metallurgy and materials science and related disciplines. At the time, the subject of 'dislocation concepts' was new and exciting, and it has remained a core discipline. The book has been an important undergraduate text all over the world. The reader should note that the dislocations discussed in the book are very important in understanding the mechanical properties of metals and ceramics, they should not, however, be confused with the activities in the A and E departments of hospitals!

My second book, *An Introduction to Composite Materials*, was first published in 1981 and reprinted six times before a second edition was published in 1997, in collaboration with a colleague skilled in new aspects of a field of science and engineering which was developing rapidly. The book was part of a series of advanced texts devoted to solid state physics initiated by Cambridge University Press, who invited three internationally recognised scientists to select relevant subject areas and authors, and to act as advisory editors. As with *The Introduction to Dislocations,* the original book was based on a final year university course which was also relevant to the development of the application of composite materials in a wide range of engineering developments from aeroplanes and motor vehicles to buildings and medical applications.

The initiative for my next two books occurred after I formally retired from the University of Cambridge and were closely related to two widely different personal interests. Leaving Cambridge, we moved back to the North, close to Liverpool. We built a bungalow less than a mile from our previous home in Heswall. We could see the Irish Sea and had spectacular views of the Dee Estuary and the Welsh Hills. This was our seventh new home and we called it 'Lanyork VII'. The number is obvious, and the name derives from our roots. I was born in Lancashire and Pauline was born in Yorkshire. We renewed all our friendships and I set up research facilities in both the University of Liverpool and the University of Cambridge. Although all our seven homes were new-builds I had no intention of resigning myself to dedicating my remaining years to gardening. After all, I had designed seven new gardens and transformed them into 'manageable' easy to maintain amenities. Things were not so easy for Pauline. In her later years in Cambridge, her health had caused some concern. Two days after the carpets had been laid in Lanyork VII she returned to Papworth and Addenbrooke's Hospitals in Cambridge for a triple heart by-pass. Although she now must take nineteen pills a day, she has survived for over twenty-five years and is the chief carer of her husband of sixty-four years, who is registered severely sight impaired and has not driven on roads or fairways for well over three years.

The two books I wrote after returning to Heswall are significantly different to Books 1 and 2. They remind me of many of the activities I enjoyed when my sight was good. Both books, although very different in their subject matter, are illustrated by hundreds of fascinating images. It will be difficult to explain the subjects adequately, but I will try to do so now.

The third book is called *Fractography: Observing, Measuring and Interpreting Fracture Surface Topography*. The subject embraces many aspects of my research, professional interests and career, and it was published in 1999. As it seems unlikely that the subject of fractography will mean much to my readers, I would like to describe a simple example that may offer an insight into what it is about and may just give some clues for those struggling with it. I must take you to the north coast of Northern Ireland to see the world-famous geological feature called Giant's Causeway. About 50 million years ago, volcanic activity resulted in the flow of molten lava across the land creating a layer of molten rock a few metres thick. As the lava slowly cooled, it solidified and became solid rock. When it cooled further, the rock shrinkage caused stresses which developed into an array of cracks, rather like the cracks that form in drying mud. The gradual cooling over a long period of time caused the layer to become a vast, densely packed collection of vertical parallel columns in a well-defined pattern. The vertical columns are approximately 0.5 metres in width, with cross-sections close to a hexagon in shape. Eventually, the columns split into a series of 'biscuit shaped' blocks stacked on top of each other and about 50cm tall.

Today, the Giant's Causeway consists of about forty thousand closely spaced columns of varying height with some reaching 25 metres high, jutting out of the cliff face as if they were stepping stones creeping into the sea. Visitors are free to walk and clamber over the tops of the columns. Each face of the blocks or 'biscuits' was formed by fracture. The cracking has produce characteristic patterns on the fracture surface from which it is possible to determine where the crack started and the way in which it grew. The Giant's Causeway is one of nature's best examples of the world of fractures which has captured my attention throughout my professional life.

The opportunity to do personal research in two outstanding university departments with state of the art research facilities and libraries, and best of all, with high-quality academic research staff, was a real privilege. My objective was to do personal research on important topics relating to the many scientific problems I had been fascinated by over the previous forty years. I set my sights on finding evidence to link the processes involved in the fracture of materials of all kinds, from metals to complex rocks, the conditions under which separation and failure of these materials had occurred and the nature and form of the fracture.

In this work, there were many opportunities for photographic studies and I searched many sources around the world to expand my knowledge. Thus, for example, I pursued American friends and colleagues who had done many important fractographic studies. I spent a month exploring some brilliant work at the US Naval Research Laboratories in Washington (after clearing security, of course!). I spent time searching for cracks in the sewers of San Diego, California to help resolve an insurance claim about the failure of the glass reinforced composites used to line the sewers. Nearer to home, I gathered important data from German scientists. And still closer, I went to the Inner Hebrides to study the superb columns of fractured basalt in Fingal's Cave on the uninhabited island of Staffa. The unique structure of the sea cave generates the acoustics which inspired the composer Felix Mendelsohn in 1829 to write the overture *'The Hebrides' opus 26,* (also known as *Fingal's Cave Overture*). The structure of the columns which form Fingal's Cave is similar to those of the Giant's Causeway. So much so, that according to the legend, the Giant's Causeway was built by the Irish giant Fionn MacCumhaill (Finn MacCool), from Gaelic mythology, who was challenged to a fight by the Scottish giant Bernadine. Fionn built the causeway across to Scotland so that he could fight the Scot!

We had a special bonus from our visit to this wild island – the puffins were in residence and they don't stay long. However, the really hard work was done in university laboratories with detailed studies of the intricate patterns on the fracture surfaces to interpret parameters such as the direction and speed of crack growth. I enjoyed an endless succession of martensitic moments – science is such good fun. Even more challenging is writing up one's finding for publication. I was very pleased when Cambridge University Press agreed to publish my book. It is a beautiful book, and you can read it in Japanese as well!

My last book was of a different kind and created a new challenge for my eyesight, even though my real eye problems were not evident when I started to develop it. I was walking in a beautiful country lane in North Wales on a balmy Sunday morning enjoying the hedgerows filled with wildflowers. In the middle of a field on a hillside, I saw a very large circle-headed cross which had been carved out of brown-red sandstone. The cross displayed complex patterns which I later discovered had been carved over a thousand years previously by people with Celtic and Viking connections. I was fascinated by the patterns. This was the start of a four-year project to understand the way that patterns of this kind are created, particularly in relation to the geometrical methods used in their construction.

I soon discovered, after numerous visits to local and national libraries, that patterns of this kind decorate hundreds of Celtic crosses all over the United Kingdom and Ireland. Fortunately, someone associated with the University of Liverpool had collected many books and manuscripts on Celtic work, and these were stored in the Special Collections Section of the library. I noted that there was a very close connection between the structure of the patterns on stone crosses and those used to ornament Celtic documents of the sixth and seventh centuries, as on the world-famous manuscripts associated with the *Book of Kells* and the *Book of Durrow*, held in Trinity College Dublin, and the *Lindisfarne Gospels* which are now kept at the British Library.

Pauline and I travelled hundreds of miles all over Wales, England, Scotland and Ireland to view and photograph a variety of stone crosses and books displaying a great range of brilliant patterns. It was a wonderful experience.

The real challenge, having collected hundreds of photographs and wrestled with the attempts of earlier archaeologists and artists, was to work out the detailed geometrical procedures of the patterns. Without the benefit of drawing in the present book, it is difficult to explain what is involved and how complicated the procedures are. Looking at the ornamentation of the Lindisfarne Gospels creates a sense of pure wonder and amazement that the monks could produce such fine and precise detail in a tiny cell in a monastery surrounded by sea.

The analysis demonstrates that all the patterns are based on a simple geometrical approach that requires the sole use of a straight edge and a set of dividers. Here's a simple first task: try yourself to divide a straight line into two equal parts using only a set of compasses.

The extent of the research required to produce the results and understanding necessary to write the textbooks three and four described above, the study of crack geometry and the details of the patterns in Celtic art, made severe demands on my eyesight and, at times, was accompanied by noticeable discomfort. I recall asking my GP and optometrist many times if they thought this eye strain could cause permanent damage. Incidentally, this was a few years before any evidence was observed in clinics and I was unaware of any resolution issues in my eyes, in fact, I thought I had been blessed with very good sight and definition.

Many topographic studies of fractures require very high-resolution observations to determine the finest details of the fracture surface. At times, knowledge of this detail is essential for an understanding of the fracture processes and I used many sophisticated 'state of the art' high-resolution facilities: optical microscopes, electron microscopes and scanning electron microscopes, to determine the intimate detail of the way the cracks grew in minute samples of fractured material. The detail can be critical, sometimes at the scale of the dimensions of individual atoms – remember one atom is about 10^{-8} cm.

The need for good eyesight was of a different kind for the illustrations I developed for my book on Celtic art. The decorative art created in the monasteries on the manuscripts produced in the seventh to 10th centuries had a very precise geometrical detail. Part of my research required extensive analysis of the geometrical methods used by the early artists. To do this, I used a sophisticated computer graphics programme which involved using the simple Euler based procedures that were first described by the Greeks over two thousand years ago. Use of computer graphics can make complex procedures relatively simple, however, some designs require an intensity of observation which can be demanding on concentration and eyesight.

Apart from the problems associated with eye strain, these two examples clearly demonstrate that the nature of the work required for this research would now be impossible for me. Another, more subtle aspect is relevant, which simply stated is the transfer of words and thoughts in the mind to a hard copy of text when writing a book. The size of this challenge is closely dependent on the level and nature of sight loss, which in my own case is deteriorating all the time. I wonder what it will be like, if and when, I come to the end of this book.

One of the obvious means of brain-to-text transfer is dictation. In work and with sight, I had no difficulty dictating to my secretary straightforward letters and brief reports. With today's technology, I could dictate directly to my computer (though to be honest, it would help to have learnt to touch type) and then ask the computer to read back what I had dictated. This can usually be done automatically, or alternatively by printing a hard copy and then listening to it with a 'reading' machine. Making corrections is like asking the secretary to do it again. For important letters etc., which I needed to think about, I would normally write these out in longhand before asking my secretary to type a draft. The process of fine-tuning the content is very important and can be demanding, particularly for writing books.

Here one reaches another hurdle when vision is almost impossible, and the already complex task becomes more problematical, without the ability to rapidly scan and rescan the written word with the eye. I am reminded of one of my early sessions at the Wirral Society for the Blind and Partially Sighted (WSBPS) in Birkenhead, when I sat in with a man going through the steps of trying to learn Braille. The challenge of learning braille is huge, not singularly because the eyes can't see the myriad of tiny elevated dots, but because the brain must learn such a complex new task of relating all the varying combinations of dots to a letter of the alphabet, a number, or one of the fourteen punctuation marks in the English language. It becomes an exercise in the ability to transfer tactile information into a visualization, and the memory and comprehension of this information. In turn, the latter part of the mechanism i.e. memory and comprehension, takes me back and reminds me of when I went to primary school and the way we learnt to read, and the repetitive chanting by the class of words on the blackboard. Or delving even further back, to childhood when we didn't do very much at all but listen to mum!

So, how could I overcome the hurdle of not being able to scan and rescan my written words when writing my book? And without this ability, how could I then continue to formulate the text, to adjust and edit until satisfied with the result? It seemed inevitable that I would have to learn new skills as quickly as my sight was failing. I was already competent on the use of computers, having used them for many tasks since their conception for work-related topics and then in the 1980s when the personal computer became the commonplace technology with the Commodore, Amstrad and IBM computers being the forerunners. My touch-typing skills, however, were somewhat lacking. Like most of my generation of computer users, we simply used a couple of fingers and a slower speed to type as required. Only the trained typist or secretary had true touch-typing skills in the 1980s. Nowadays, the millennial generation and younger, like my granddaughters, tell me that touch typing for the computer is taught at school. There are plenty of 'high-tech' technologies such as computer voice over, computerized dictation, Siri, Alexa – artificial intelligence, etc., which can help the visually impaired connect with the outside world. I tried to utilize them all, but each one required an immense learning curve. Computers developed rapidly and today are a far cry from the original binary-based programming, with Apple and Microsoft locked in a perpetual race to make their operating systems easier, quicker, and foolproof whilst remaining secure. All the while, the relatively simple skills of touch typing morphed into predictive text, windows, swiping left, right, up, down and a plethora of other hand *movements and signals* to activate keys, mice, and touchscreens. It all seems very simple when one looks at one's children and grandchildren who are instantly playing with remarkable ease on iPads and iPhones. But surely, this is a result of having played with these devices for hours and hours!

These computer skills must be learnt, and the key here is finding a good teacher, listening and working at it with lots of patience, which brings me back to the difficulties of learning braille. Any new skill on the computer is inevitably hampered by a deterioration of sight. We all learn differently. There are visual, aural, physical, verbal or linguistic and logical learners. There are social learners and solitary ones. Some use a different combination of styles to learn in differing circumstances, whilst others can develop their abilities in their less dominant styles. Traditional schooling used (and some still do) mainly linguistic and logical styles of teaching, and certainly, my early memories of school days are learning through books with repetition, reinforcement and review. Perhaps this is why the ability to scan and rescan my draft text was so important to me? Initially, I learnt to use the voice-over facility on the computer to read back to me a phrase, a paragraph or a page which I had painstakingly typed. This was helpful as the difficulty of reading even the enlarged print on a computer screen became more pronounced. The commands had to be learnt, the sequence of keys mastered to activate voice-over or to switch it off when Mr Voiceover just kept on reading! Also, the aural style of learning needed reactivating and cultivating, teaching myself to listen carefully, visualize, memorize and action. One of the methods for asking voiceover to read part of a text on the computer is to highlight the section and press command keys to activate the voiceover. The challenges were many: highlighting the right section, finding the command keys, listening intently and then finding the spot where the correction or addition needed to be made. Many a time, words carefully chosen and laboriously written vanished as I inadvertently hit the delete command keys in error. Where was my secretary?

It was at this point that I decided to enlist the help of a sighted-person. It was either that or give up and abandon a book halfway through. Fortunately, when I posed the question to one of my daughters, Karen, almost twelve months ago whilst walking through the beautiful surroundings of Burton Mere Wetlands, a nature reserve on the Dee Estuary straddling the border between Cheshire, England and Flintshire, Wales and run by the Royal Society for the Protection of Birds, she agreed to help. Some years previously, Karen had introduced me to Audible books as a 'low-technology' means to continue 'reading' books when the printed word became an arduous trial rather than the invigorating pleasure it should be. I also invested in another piece of technology, the Text to Speech Scanner. This excellent piece of equipment will scan and audibly read back almost any typed document, letters, bills, appointment cards etc. and has allowed me to set up a system whereby I could print out sections of my draft writings, scan them and hear them read back to me repeatedly. Part of the cycle was working. To overcome the progressively increasing difficulties of typing, we found that, when Karen came over to the house or even, on occasion over the telephone, I could dictate to her and she would type directly to the word processing program. When the 90-mile round trip for Karen was not possible, I have reverted to putting my thoughts down in an age-old manner with pen and paper. I am unable to read them back and must wait for Karen to transcribe them into printed text. And so, the circle completes.

As I reflect on the labour of trying to learn new skills whilst my eyesight was deteriorating, I am reminded of the law graduation ceremony for one of my granddaughters at the University of Leeds last year. The email we received from her following the event mentioned how amazed she was that the address had been given by a former law graduate of the University, Colin McKenzie Low, Lord Colin Low of Dalston. He was receiving an honorary degree from the University that day for his work in Disability Law. What had amazed her the most was that Lord Low had given the address whilst reading from a Braille display machine. The content of the address may have been a little wasted on her as she was fascinated by how he was using this machine, his fingers flying across the silent keys: "It was just like a laptop, but he played it like a piano!", she commented.

A little research tells us that Lord Colin Low, born in Scotland in 1942, has been blind since he was three years old. He has been a lifelong supporter of human rights particularly with respect to disabilities, held the chair of the Royal National Institute for the Blind and in 2006 received a lifelong peerage at the House of Lords. In his maiden speech on 21 November, 2006, to the House of Lords, he drew attention to blindness being one of the severest disabilities, and the urgent need for change to help those afflicted with their 'normal' lives, and these were his words on the rapidly advancing technological world: *"Technology is a great force for inclusion, and we can now access much information which was formerly a closed book. But if the needs of the blind are not kept in mind when designing new devices, it can be just as great a force for exclusion. Try operating an iPod, a touchscreen, or a digital radio with your eyes closed. Most worrying of all, unless someone comes up with an electronic program guide which is accessible PDQ, digital switchover is going to mean digital switch-off so far as visually impaired people are concerned."*

One can't help wondering whether the challenges I have faced writing this book would have been less had

I mastered braille whilst my vision was still adequate, and I was not so reliant on it, and whether with the increasing incidence of AMD and other ageing sight-related disabilities it would be beneficial to increase the availability of braille learning facilities. I have been told that a report commissioned by the Royal National Institute for the Blind (RNIB) in 2009, "*Braille in the 21st century: opportunities, benefits, and challenges for adults with acquired sight loss*", looked at some of the difficulties with learning braille as an adult. Canvassing opinion from teachers, services associated with sight impairment and adults who had learnt or tried to learn braille it drew many conclusions. Notably, it highlighted that older people often find learning braille more difficult than younger people, as frequently they are anxious about learning new skills and may have diminished touch sensitivity. And whilst it agreed, that one solution of using 'low-tech' equipment such as audiobooks matched or was better than braille in some aspects of information access, it quoted some comments from those visually impaired who had mastered braille, saying braille had made them feel 'less passive', helped them 'maintain independence', that they 'didn't retain information from audible means', and that 'reading through braille, I can give my own interpretation to the words, which was not possible with recorded books'.

Anyway, I comfort myself with the thought that there is plenty of time for this book and at the end of the day it doesn't matter if it is published. But the writing has been interesting and worthwhile, and it fills time in a much more effective way than sitting watching the television!

Chapter 5

Losing Sight

It is nearly eighteen years since my first visit to the eye clinic at my local hospital, Arrowe Park. It is only three or four miles away and only five years since I was diagnosed with wet and dry AMD, Age-related Macular Degeneration. Sixteen years ago, I was almost totally unaware of the wide range of ailments that cause poor vision. I am now aware that there are numerous, and often very distressing eye conditions and that the eye saga for each varies widely from patient to patient – each story is unique. Within my own group of conditions, identified broadly as AMD and, rather more subtly, classified as conditions in which there is damage to the macula of the retina of the eye, there are many sufferers. Thirty years ago, a group of sufferers and well-wishers formed a voluntary organisation now called The Macular Society, which is dedicated to supporting people affected by a macular disease and raising funds to support the research seeking to understand the intricacies of the condition and find routes for healing and care.

In telling my story, I am fully aware that my knowledge and understanding of all things to do with eyes is very limited. Apart from some sixth form optics, I know little about Ophthalmology and similar comments can be made about all the other skills required to investigate and treat patients with poor eyes. I can claim to have had some experience of the relationship between modern materials, science and engineering and the powerful benefits that can be derived from interactions between medical sciences and material sciences. For many years, I was chairman of a government research fund committee responsible for allocating government funds, and some of my research has involved problems like the development of vascular implants, hip replacements and dental fillings.

My first visit to the eye clinic was triggered by visits to the local opticians in 1998 – 2000 when I was still in Cambridge. I was needing some magnification for reading particularly for my left eye. I had been very active with microscopy and although the opticians didn't seem to agree, I suspected this was a factor in explaining my sore eyes at the end of the day.

In May 2000, my Heswall optician referred me to Arrowe Park Hospital because the Snellen alphabet test showed a weakness of the left eye and evidence of a blind spot in the top right-hand corner of the eye. Eye pressures were said to be normal at 160 (there were no units stated and these must have been different to current units used). A field of vision scan was not available but the consultant, after waving a pointed pencil in front of my eye, detected some local blindness, but only hinted at this possibility and the presence of some glaucoma. Later this possibility was withdrawn and the alternative recourse of damage to the optic nerve was suggested. I was prescribed half an aspirin to thin my blood.

At this stage, I was discharged because there was little evidence of any further changes. Four years later, at a routine visit to the optician to check on my reading glasses, I reported that in very low light conditions I saw a weak dark cloud in my left eye. My eye pressures were normal despite glaucoma being suspected. Visits to Arrowe Park hospital over the next year, 2005 – 06, included a detailed examination of the back of my eyes, which were inconclusive, and suggestions were directed to blood supply problems to the optic nerve. Once again, I was discharged.

During optician's tests in 2008, I reported the dark shadows in my eyes after being in the bright sunshine and a significant deterioration of the sight in my right eye. The optician said there were 'drusens', yellow deposits which form under the retina, suggesting dry macular degeneration. My eye problems were of a different kind almost a month later when a hard, rigid twig pierced my eye in a gardening accident. I was admitted to the Accident and Emergency department, and the tear in my eye was repaired with stitches. The doctor confirmed the presence of drusens and advised the use of an *Amsler grid*, a diagnostic tool to monitor a person's central field of vision using a series of vertical and horizontal lines. Straight lines are good, wavy or distorted lines are not.

In November 2009, another Arrowe Park consultant and my optician were struggling with a clear diagnosis of my eyes, seemingly unable to distinguish between glaucoma, AMD and cataracts. After pressing for a clearer picture, I was invited to read the literature of Harvard Medical School to try and resolve a possible diagnosis of low-pressure glaucoma. So, how about a brain tumour explanation, which could be checked out with an MRI scan? This showed that there was a *'periventricular* white matter hyperintensity, or high signal, consistent with an ischaemic change'. All this was followed by a series of other tests. However, no connection was found relating to the various nose operations I had many years earlier to relieve nasal congestion. Perhaps my feelings of confusion are familiar to other readers who have experienced the blind alley of an undiagnosed condition, elusive in its presentation and interpretation despite all best efforts. The mass of medical terminology, although sketchy in its identification of a specific condition, left me with a mountain of questions and ambiguities to fathom; a science professor's headache. Only when a problem is identified and recognised can any forward progress be made in treatment, management and acceptance, and I admit to finding the unknown a personal challenge, and to spending many hours searching the internet.

Over the next two years, I had regular tests in hospital and at the opticians. Vague signs of macular degeneration and cataracts were mentioned, and my eye pressures remained at a steady 11 to 12. I was given another copy of the *Amsler grid*. Amongst some of my friends, the problems of deteriorating sight were being discussed. One friend was starting to have injections for wet AMD, and another was waiting to have a distressing operation to reduce a growth close to his pituitary gland, which was thought to be pressing on his optic nerve. Remarkably, my vision was still very good, and my lifestyle, interests and activities were unaffected by eye difficulties apart from the need to increase the strength of my glasses for reading, photography and art pursuits.

In November 2012 all this changed. My left eye displayed many changes, and the telegraph poles altered from straight to wavy lines. All images were blurred and the contrast within the images decreased, particularly in darker conditions. I was very conscious that I couldn't focus with my left eye. Since the optician was on an extended holiday I had to wait for an appointment. Eventually, the optician had little hesitation in concluding that these symptoms could be accounted for by the onset of AMD. A fax message to Arrowe Park eye clinic resulted in an appointment within eight days and an apology from the optician. Numerous tests were undertaken to establish that I had wet AMD in my left eye and dry AMD in my right eye.

I think it would be useful at this juncture to pause for a moment to consider the normal form of the eye. It's a very complex structure and I don't suggest that I understand more than the basics of the make-up of the eye. At our meetings at The Macular Society, we always have a large wall poster diagram of the eye on display, not to learn piecemeal but to keep in mind the main structures to allow a better understanding of the issues that might be dis- cussed by the speakers and in breakaway groups of members. It seems a very popular idea with the members as there are plenty of new terms, words and concepts to absorb and bring into focus with the many facets of macular, and indeed a host of other eye diseases. I admit to having had the help of my assistant, Karen, to collate the details and hopefully put into words a description of our poster. So, here is some science as I understand it:

The retina sits at the back of the inside of the eye sphere and is made up of two main layers. The inner layer is made of 'seeing' cells called 'rods' and 'cones' which react to light and send electric signals via the optic nerve to the brain. The outer layer – the retinal pigment epithelium (RPE) – is a layer of cells behind the rods and cones.

The RPE is very important as it helps to nourish and support the 'seeing cells' and acts as a filter to keep harmful substances away from the very sensitive rods and cones. The macula is a small area of the retina about 5mm in diameter, and it is here that the rods and cones are most densely packed and where the central vision is formed. In the middle of the macula is an area called the fovea, which only contains cone cells and it is responsible for the pin-point central vision. Finally, there is a layer of blood vessels between the retina and the outer, firm layer of the eye, the sclera. These tiny blood vessels of the choroid bring oxygen and nutrients to the retina.

Age-related macular degeneration (AMD) is an increasingly common ailment that occurs when the cells in the macula begin to degenerate with advancing years. The most common form is dry AMD. In this type, it is the cells of the outer layer (RPE) of the macula which gradually become thin and degenerate. As these cells are crucial for the health of the rods and cones, these also degenerate and die. Not only do the cells of the RPE fail to take enough nutrients to the rods and cones, but they are also unable to clear waste and by-products. As a result, tiny abnormal deposits called *drusens* develop under the retina. It is a gradual process and usually takes several years for the vision to become seriously affected.

The other form is wet AMD, also called neovascular or exudative AMD. The difference is that in wet AMD, in addition to the outer layer (RPE) of the retina degenerating, there is the growth of abnormal blood vessels from the choroid at the back of the eye. These vessels then grow under and into the macula. The new abnormal blood vessels may then leak blood or fluid. This can damage the rods and cone cells, and cause distortion and scarring of the macula leading to further vision loss. Wet AMD distorts the central vision more significantly; it can cause severe visual loss over quite a short period of time. Very occasionally, a large bleed can result in very sudden vision loss within hours or days. It is not known why there is this increase and growth of abnormal blood vessels, although it is thought that waste products or a shortage of oxygen may be involved.

To identify wet AMD, the retina is examined using fluorescent angiography, a technique in which a dye is injected into a vein in the hand and the dyes then pass to the eye. It fluoresces when viewed using a microscope, allowing the pattern and pathology of the blood vessels to be determined.

Returning to my story, we can see that the news of my diagnosis was not good or welcome, and in the words of the Speaker of the House of Common, "The 'Ayes' have it".

Wet AMD is usually treated by injections, directly into the globe of the eye, of medications such as bevacizumab (Avastin), anti-vascular endothelial growth factor or anti-VEGF. This may help to stop the growth of new blood vessels by blocking the effects of growth signals or hormones the body sends. Often the injections are given every four weeks to maintain the beneficial effect of the medication. In some instances, there may be a partial recovery of vision as the blood vessels shrink and the fluid under the retina absorbs, allowing retinal cells to regain some function.

There is no specific therapeutic intervention to treat the more common dry AMD yet, although research continues to develop, and the new intraocular lens system may eventually offer hope for advanced dry AMD.

I had my first eye injection eight days later. The clinic was very busy, and many patients were treated. One of my friends had already had injections and had told me all the steps involved. Apart from the natural apprehension, the procedure is bearable. A nurse put drops on the outer edge of the eye to provide anaesthetic to minimise pain and provide some sterilisation. The doctor covered the upper part of my face before inserting the needle into the side of the eyeball. A slight pressure feeling occurred in the eye as a liquid was injected. Five minutes later, I slid off the table relieved and went home. It was all over, thank goodness. My next injection was given four weeks later. The doctor seemed disappointed in my report of the changes in the eye during this time, but I had no idea of what was expected and couldn't make any assessment. I had seven injections in about a year and formed the impression, from the response of the medics, that they had not resulted in a favourable outcome.

The next big trauma occurred in July 2013. I awoke to find that I had lost all vision in 80% of my left eye; it was totally black. I made many telephone calls to try and get an appointment at the eye clinic. Eventually, my present hospital consultant saw me and took control of both the AMD and glaucoma conditions, although he was not optimistic that anything could be done, and I was rather unwilling to accept any of the possible approaches that were suggested to remove the massive haemorrhage which had caused the black-out. A conference was called for three days' time. My daughter, a specialist in child autism, insisted on travelling from her home near Derby, not to be an eye doctor but to hold my hand. After much consideration, the consultant decided to try and remove the blood from the eye by a complex sequence of procedures the following day. I trusted him to do his best. The procedures were long and uncomfortable, and sadly the outcome was not successful. Words like 'neovascular AMD, left intravitreal injection and intraocular C3F8 *tamponade*' were used, but barely understood by me.

A few days later, in-depth observations were made on my right eye to assess its condition with respect to wet AMD. I was advised that, in the future, I should contact the hospital immediately on noticing any signs of wet AMD.

The massive haemorrhage incident suggested to me that the prospect of a progressive deterioration of my sight was likely and that I had no timescales. My mind, or was it my brain, then moved on to the actions I should take to help me, with the limited sight I had, to prepare for this almost inevitable event. Some of the remaining chapters in this book may give some ideas of what I did. An immediate reaction was to think about the implications. I like to walk alone to think. I followed one of my favourite paths across the fields on rolling hillsides and through farmyards. I enjoyed the sounds of the birds and the smell of the farm animals. I knew that the birds weren't singing louder, but I was more aware of them and reflected on my school essay of seventy years ago: Which is the more precious, sight or hearing?

So, following the events of July 2013, I had regular visits for check-ups. The idea of second opinions was not pursued, for what I considered to be good reasons, and at every visit, my sight was monitored with a field of vision scan and the Snellen alphabet chart. The latter seemed to give a reliable indication of the general position. Using my left eye, I couldn't even see the chart, never mind the letters on the chart – and still can't. I had a small amount of navigational skill, so I usually missed lampposts even when my right eye was closed. In July 2013, my right eye could read almost all the letters down to the bottom row. I could see very well with one eye.

One of my enjoyments that I had no problem with was playing golf and I continued to play regularly with my friends. However, I started to notice that, after I had played a few holes, my heartbeat which was usually perfectly regular, began to develop an irregular beat. This became the new feature of my eye saga and I now know to call this irregularity atrial fibrillation.

The onset of atrial fibrillation produced an unresolved digression in the eye saga. The heart specialists decided that the appropriate treatment was a daily dose of Warfarin, originally produced as a rat poison. In low doses it affects the behaviour of the blood which, in layman's terms, is said to allow the blood to flow more easily through the heart and reduce the likelihood of the formation of clots or plaques on the walls of the heart, which in turn could break away and move to the brain or lungs and lead to a stroke or pulmonary embolism. This diagnosis and treatment coincided with discussions in the eye clinic about the observation that blood was escaping into the back of the eye leading to wet AMD. It occurred to me that the Warfarin treatment could affect the blood flow in the back of the eye and aggravate the process of AMD. With evidence from Google searches by my medically trained children, I talked this dilemma through with the consultants involved without resolution except for the bleak conclusion, or one could say the choice of, 'to continue with Warfarin and minimize the prospect of death by a stroke, or risk further advances in the loss of my sight'. The dilemma is apparent between the treatment of one condition and the outcome of another.

Things quietened down as far as the hospital was concerned in the following three years. Several routine tests indicated some deterioration in the right eye and I was aware of this because my sight was getting worse with poor resolution, greyer images, darker landscapes and the field of vision tests showed that the top two segments were blind. As if searching for a needle in a haystack, I had a CT scan and some blood tests, but there wasn't much, if any, feedback. I was offered the services of optometrists who sought to find hand-held magnifying devices, but they only gave limited improvements. The eye pressures remained stable between 11 and 13. An upgraded machine was used to examine the back of my eye by the field of vision technician. I had emergency tests when I became aware of wiggly lines in the right eye and an emergency consultant decided that I was severely, partially sighted. Finally, in April 2017, following another set of retina photographs and Snellen test, the ophthalmic consultant was prompted to tell me that there was real evidence of a serious deterioration of my right eye and that it was caused by a form of dry AMD for which there was no treatment. We then discussed cataract operations and the possibility of approaching the London Eye Hospital for a lens implant treatment, which gives me a 'hole-in-the-head' feeling.

Part of me regrets recalling this sorry saga of loss of sight and I little doubt that the downhill deterioration will continue. I feel supported by the staff at the eye clinic and by a host of family and friends. As if signalling a wider awareness of my sight difficulties, various agencies within the hospital and other groups became involved in helping me with the problems of making the best use of my limited sight. Their help has been generous, and they keep regular contact with me. I have been offered various means of managing to keep walking, navigational skills, training with computers and other electrical devices, and I have attended various meetings at which a wide range of gadgets are displayed. I can now make a cup of tea without pouring hot water all over the kitchen thanks to a clever liquid level device. Every little helps! I must admit though that I don't find any comfort in the knowledge that there are many people who are struggling with much worse conditions than my own.

There is good news that solutions are being found for many eye problems and that there are many people who have benefited from the treatment and care offered at eye clinics. Recently, I sat with an elderly lady in the clinic who was waiting, as I was, to be picked up by her car driver to be driven home. She had lost the sight in her left eye to AMD but had had a remarkable improvement in the sight in her right eye after five injections. "Great news! I will be able to watch TV!" she said.

At the start of the New Year, I had a review of the state of my eyes after another round of routine tests and eye photos. The eye pressures were eight and 11, I couldn't see all the alphabet letters in my left eye and could barely detect the movement of a hand in front of the eye. My right eye struggled to read halfway down the eye chart. The eye photographs indicated a small deterioration in the condition of my eyes since the last photographs a few weeks previously. I pressed the doctor for an assessment of the prospects of retaining sufficient sight to navigate around objects in the future. It was rather unfair of me, but I persuaded myself that I should not plan by thought and deed for complete blindness. Nevertheless, I realise that further deterioration of sight was likely and that there are already sight issues to be added to the sorry tale I have told so far. I am on the waiting list for a cataract removal from my left eye and recently, I have had several episodes of Charles Bonnet Syndrome.

It is said that of the hundreds of thousands of people in the UK who suffer from sight loss or visual impairment that is approaching blindness, over 20 – 30% experience a form of visual 'hallucinations' first described by a young natural scientist in 1760. Charles Bonnet wrote an essay describing the 'visions' that his maternal grandfather, a retired magistrate, was experiencing as he lost his sight in the later years of his life. Many years later, the condition that Charles Bonnet had noted was attributed to him and called Charles Bonnet Syndrome (CBS). Today this condition is recognised as the occurrence of phantom visions in people living with some form of acquired vision loss, who are otherwise mentally healthy.

The descriptions of the phantom visions or images experienced can vary widely from person to person. They can be clearly defined pictures or abstract, geometrical shapes. They can have quirky irregularities such as faces superimposed on solid objects or buildings of a bygone era interspersed within a current day image. Often, particularly when first experienced, the phantom visions can be startling and even frightening, yet despite this, the sufferer is frequently amazed at the detail within the images. Sadly, although Charles Bonnet Syndrome has been known about for a long time, there seems to be little acknowledgement or understanding of the condition by medical and health-care practitioners, which can leave the sufferer feeling bewildered. Since few people who experience these symptoms are likely to discuss them with family members, friends, or physicians, for fear of being misunderstood, it has been suggested that the actual number of sufferers may be significantly higher.

Over the years, long before my eye problems began, I wondered about the workings of the brain. My searches for understanding have been frustrated by the sheer complexity of the brain and the range of technical words used to describe its anatomy and explain its workings, which are convoluted to a scholar of medicine and baffling to a layman. Indeed, one of my highly intelligent nephews abandoned his medical studies because his mild dyslexia was so challenged by the myriad of anatomical words that it impaired his medical understanding.

A few of my brain cells, I don't know which ones and if I did I wouldn't tell you, were tugged by a description of Charles Bonnet Syndrome at the Macular Society conference three or four years ago. My thirst for knowledge took me to Wikipedia and I studied a video lecture by the world-famous neurologist, Oliver Sacks, who was talking to a group of American medical students about the Charles Bonnet Syndrome, which leads to incredible visual experiences that many people find very disturbing. He talked about his patients who suffer from Charles Bonnet Syndrome, who have described their 'hallucinations' to him in a very clear and lucid way. He emphasised that all the patients were aware that the 'hallucinations' were not real, and that they were unencumbered by any of the other senses, such as smell or hearing.

So, when I met people in my own Macular Society group who said they were affected, to some extent I could chat with them about this problem. It was some months later that my own phantom images invaded my experience. My hallucinations, although at times very varied and transient, are frequently geometrical in nature and as I sit in my study, dictating these words to Karen, I can look across to the wall, on which I know, in reality there is a simple painting against a plain, white background, and see, or perceive, a vision of a network of blue grid lines rather like a giant piece of graph paper. At other times, the vision might be of a ten-storey high building with an architecture completely out of character with the detached, four-bedroom house that I watched being built across the street from our house. Even today, looking over my daughter's shoulder as she typed, a new vision appeared. The text was in upper case letters, when in fact it was all lower case. Mind-blowing, as I am unable to see text with that sort of definition normally. Where do these images come from? What controls their nature and appearance?

Charles Bonnet Syndrome, also sometimes referred to as 'phantom vision' syndrome, was first noted over two hundred years ago, and the answers to the causes are still some way off, which suggests there is scope for extensive scientific exploration, already referred to in Oliver Sachs' video. However, it is reassuring to know that the presence of these pseudo-hallucinations does not indicate an unstoppable decline of memory, dementia or senility. Current research is advancing to find an alternative treatment to the use of drugs, which only helps a few sufferers and can also cause serious side effects. Indeed, in recent months, the subject of CBS has gradually been finding its way into conversation, and organisations such as Esme's Umbrella, a campaign group working towards greater awareness of Charles Bonnet Syndrome, are raising its profile on various media outlets and forums. A study at Newcastle University is underway to look at the use of transcranial direct current stimulation (tDCS) and has been seeking willing participants. To help understand this approach, the Lighthouse Guild, a charitable organisation based in New York providing healthcare for the visually impaired and blind, explains the 'phantom vision' associated with CBS as follows: *The cause of this disorder is thought to be a misfire in the brain similar to the neurological mix-up that occurs in patients with phantom limb syndrome. As vision wanes, the brain continues to interpret visual imagery in the absence of corresponding visual input, just as it sometimes continues to process pain signals from a limb that's no longer there.*

The Newcastle study uses transcranial direct current stimulation (whatever that is) in which a mild electric current is passed between two or more pads on the head. It is hoped that this will normalise the activity in the visual system which is thought to cause the phantom visions of Charles Bonnet Syndrome. If the study is successful, the next step is to produce handheld devices enabling people to treat their hallucinations at home. There is a long way to go, but there is hope that research such as this will add a wealth of knowledge about the causes of the hallucinations. For now, the one fundamental aid to the management of this condition is the acknowledgement of it by carers, family, friends and medical staff, and the reassurance that this gives to the patient. In our household, there have been many conversations about the bears sitting at the side of my dinner plate while I try to find my sausages, the green cat who runs in through the backdoor uninvited, and my brother who pops up at the end of my bed, and I share with you, at the end of this chapter, my daughter's rather fun description of the condition.

One thought stays with me, part of the unanswerable question, will my eye condition stabilise, what will happen if it progresses, how do AMD, glaucoma, cataracts etc. plot my future, and how will I cope with further deterioration of my sight? It is more than missing lampposts or cars with wing mirrors parked alongside the pavement or even cutting up my sausages! How do people cope? A perfectly sensible question, as the medics try to find answers and alleviate the present symptoms. Even as I put the finishing touches to this part of my story, there have been reports in the media of a breakthrough in the use of stem cells to treat AMD by the London Project to Cure Blindness. They have revealed that the first two patients, both severely vision-impaired with advanced AMD, have received an implanted 'patch' of stem cells over the damaged retina at the back of the eye and regained enough sight to be able to read. It is hoped that within five years this stem cell treatment could become as commonplace as cataract surgery. Great news and a great reason to keep going!

An alternative view of Charles Bonnet Syndrome – by Karen Hull

Charles Bonnet Syndrome is rather like being given a pair of virtual reality goggles pre-programmed with every image you have ever processed in your brain throughout your life. Your brain can be thought of as a multiplex cinema with millions of mini-screens which hold the images. These images can be actual, as in real things you have seen and experienced, or images you have seen in books, news-papers, films, TV, magazine, art galleries – the list is endless. Unfortunately, the software programming of the virtual reality goggles has 'gone awry' and the preloaded images are no longer neatly catalogued or sequential. You have no oper-ating manual, and someone has hidden the remote control – (it is not behind the cushion on the settee!). To add to the confusion, the battery which powers the virtual reality goggles is playing up, so that at times they are switched off and at others, for no apparent reason, they come to life; there's a trickle of electrical current from the battery and suddenly the virtual reality screen inside the goggles comes to life with random images from the back catalogue. They are jumbled and unrelated to anything you might be doing at the time, or any thought that might have preceded the battery surge. They can be in full HD technicolour or shades of grey. They can be fleeting or stay with you for longer, then just as spontaneously, the battery plays up again and they pass... for now.

The challenge for modern medicine is finding the remote control. Perhaps the multiplex cinema screens are constantly running, rather like the massive screens of Times Square, but when one knows where the remote control is, the brain tunes into the screens only when they are needed. Is this why dreams can sometimes seem very real and contextual? Is the mind re-evaluating previously stored images?

Another challenge and a far greater one would be if the clever scientists and neurosurgeons, having found the remote control, could fix the battery and make the virtual reality goggles reverse their action. Instead of seeing images already stored, the wearer would use goggles or glasses to record reality, and transfer those images, via the remote, back to the multiplex cinema in the brain, re-creating sight. Now that would be artificial intelligence at its best!

Chapter 6

Volunteering and The Macular Society

Volunteering has many clothes. Some are barely visible, others shine out like Major Generals on dress parade. Some volunteers, spend every Wednesday morning giving advice at the local Citizens Advice Bureau and others, like the founder of Microsoft Bill Gates and his wife Melinda, share their billions of dollars and encourage other wealthy individuals to do the same through The Giving Pledge, with the aim of improving global healthcare and controlling disease such as malaria, Aids, HIV and tuberculosis and of reducing extreme poverty worldwide.

Over the years I have been involved in activities which required effective volunteering (e.g. The Falkland Veterans, Rydal School, The Boys Brigade, The Samaritans) and whilst all of these involved specific tasks and skills, they didn't have a strong element of self-interest.

In about November 2012, my eyes were to change significantly and outside of my previous experience. Wet AMD was something else, and I started to seek a better idea of my prospects for the future with the now much stronger influence of the progressive loss of my sight. Many organisations offered insights and assistance to provide a whole range of practical help. There was a liaison-type link between the organisations and the hospital, which encouraged patients to make contact with a strong support group in Birkenhead called WSBPS, (the Wirral Society for Blind and Partially Sighted). This is a self-funded organisation situated in modest premises close to the centre of Birkenhead Park, an area well known for its pioneering in the design of public parks and for having been influential in the design of Central Park in New York. This facility offers social and practical facilities for the blind and partially sighted, access to a well-stocked range of aids and devices to ease the difficulties of the blind, and several courses to help and encourage individuals to utilise as many of the new skills required as possible on their hesitant path. When I visited their show area, I noticed a sign inviting volunteers to apply. I had no idea whether or not I could help, particularly as my eyesight was fading, but their need for help was evident and perhaps I could offer a year or so before my eyes gave up.

Unfortunately, I didn't get any response to my application. When I visited the centre again, I was asked if I had any particular skills to offer. I mentioned my computer interest and it was suggested that I should go and help in the computer training facility. The main problem here was that my skills are based on Apple computers whereas the computer laboratory has computers based on the Microsoft operating system. I spent an hour watching an elderly lady who was skilled at touch typing but I realised she would need many lessons to become proficient on a computer. I had a similar experience sitting with an elderly man trying to learn Braille without any previous experience. It was rather stressful, and it persuaded me that at my age Braille was unlikely to help me as my sight disappeared.

About this time, I was told about the activities of the Macular Society. Forgive me if I summarise some of the background of the Society which I learnt in the next couple of months after joining for the modest fee of £18 a year. The Society was formed in 1987 by a group of 'volunteers' seeking to give support to people suffering from diseases of the macula which is the main anatomical structure relating to central vision. The starting group have been very successful and celebrated their 30th Anniversary in 2017. The headquarters office is based in Andover, Hampshire and is led by a Chief Executive who has a professional team of around 40 staff. A set of distinguished people oversee the work of the Society led by the Chairman. In broad terms, the Society has two main objectives. First, to care for all who suffer from macular diseases – not a trivial duty considering that there are over 200,000 people in the UK who suffer from this condition. Second, to raise funds from charitable sources to fund high-level research in the field by universities and research scientists to identify and solve problems relating to macular conditions. Since 1990 the Macular Society has raised and invested £3.8 million in grants for this purpose. Of course, funds are required for many other activities that promote other key functions such as training.

The main approach to serving the needs of the membership is through a comprehensive group system which embraces the whole of the UK. There are over three hundred groups and the boundaries between each group are based on geographical and postcode factors. Each group is managed by a member of the Macular Society headquarters' team. The individual groups are almost autonomous but have some responsibilities linked to headquarters such as the promotion of the Society and the distribution of a substantial library of advertising literature and detailed information sheets relating to a whole range of macular conditions and aids.

It shouldn't be overlooked that there are many independent organisations whose objective overlap and complement those of the Macular Society and support the blind community in all sorts of ways. All are generous in their support.

When I joined the Macular Society I was allocated, based on my postcode, to the Wirral Support Group which covered the whole of the Wirral peninsula between the Mersey estuary on the east side and the Dee estuary on the west side. The area manager (Michelle Dutton) who was based in Manchester was responsible for about ten other groups in the Northwest of England. One of the important responsibilities of the area manager was to support and encourage the groups alongside initiating new ones and rebuilding those that were struggling. When I joined, the area manager was struggling to revive the Wirral Support Group which was labouring because of the demise of key members of the support team. A long-standing, faithful leader had died rather suddenly and her husband, who was serving as Treasurer, was unable to continue. The members of the Group were unable to find replacements and the Macular Society headquarters had closed the Group but kept some of the spirit of the Group alive by transferring the money in the Group's account to be released if, at some future opportunity, the Group was reactivated.

My joining the residual Wirral Group coincided with the area manager calling a meeting of any members of the Macular Society in the area to see if anything could be done. It was a dreary and depressing affair in January 2013 held at Ashville Lodge, Birkenhead, the home of the Wirral Society of Blind Partially Sighted (WSBPS). There were a few ideas about the future and a few members attended. The area manager then invited two members who had shown a limited amount of interest and had been in the Group before the previous leader had died, to reform the Wirral Group along with myself. Eventually, some progress was made.

The 'group of three' were all over eighty years old with me, 'Derek', clearly the youngest. Maurice had been a senior hospital anaesthetist, Joy had trained as an architect and had many interests in local history and was still involved with the activities of retired Mersey River Pilots, and I had retired as a Cambridge academic many years ago. With strong persuasion from the area manager, we agreed to try and form a new Group. Maurice proposed that since I had been Dean of Engineering many years ago I should be the leader. I said that if Maurice agreed to be secretary I would be leader, so it was inevitable that Joy would have to be treasurer. The area manager gave a big sigh of relief and sent a message to all past members telling them the news.

The new committee decided to follow the ways of the previous Group and have group meetings for members every two months on the last Thursday of the month with a speaker and a cup of tea. We soon discovered lots of problems. Secretary Maurice didn't have a computer and had never used one, treasurer Joy had no idea about banks and her nearest branch was two bus rides away. As for Derek, he was new to the Macular Society and had no idea of how it was organised and what it wanted to achieve.

He soon learnt that the Society had many guidance notes (rules) on the organisation and running the activities of Groups but he had some reservations which would have to be overcome. Never mind hey!! He also undertook to find suitable speakers.

The Committee decided that before every meeting the chairman should send a letter of invitation to attend the meeting to introduce information on the speaker and details of future activities. All Macular Society members and others who had been involved with macular conditions would be on the circulation list. Who would be responsible for this duty? We needed a volunteer to be membership secretary. Along came Marlene who, despite having injections for AMD and marked limitations with her vision, was willing to join the committee – without a reference. She also agreed to be responsible for circulating pamphlets and information sheets to local libraries, opticians, local hospitals, etc. on behalf of the Macular Society Headquarters.

We were determined to hold our first meeting as soon as possible and invited a friend of our secretary to give a talk. We hadn't yet decided what types of talk would be most appropriate, although the Macular Society had strong views. The few members who attended said they enjoyed his talk: 'Arrowe Park to Afghanistan'. After this experience, we decided to produce a questionnaire which was circulated to all members to give everyone an opportunity to comment. At this time, we didn't know the interest of members and it was noted that in groups, such as the Wirral Group, defined by geographical boundaries, the members may be from a range of social classes with different socio-political boundaries. The questionnaire showed that a strong majority of members favoured talks by professionals directly involved with ophthalmology and its many implications, who would be able to give our members informative lectures on topics relating to eyes.

My efforts as speaker organiser proved successful. I relied initially on many contacts within the University of Liverpool and the Liverpool hospitals. Lecture topics included nutrition, stem cells and AMD treatments. We had two lectures by the senior eye consultant at Arrowe Park Hospital which were much appreciated by many of the members who were also his patients. The attendance at the meetings steadily increased and I know the members of the committee were delighted at the May 2017 meeting. The talk by Professor Luminita Paraoan was called 'What causes Age-related Macular Degeneration?'. The meeting room in WSBPS was almost full, with an audience of over forty people. The speaker brought three of her post-doctoral workers to share the experience, and the audience enjoyed the talk immensely and asked many questions, although it was rather technical, and they wouldn't pass the examination! To encourage more participation and commu-nication between members we enjoyed a 'strawberries and cream' party in 2015 and 2016, and really pushed the boat out at the beginning of 2017 with a Burns afternoon, which was very popular. There was a full complement of all things Robbie Burns chaired by our Scottish bard, secretary Ronald, and some very generous volunteers.

After a year, our original secretary Maurice didn't resist the suggestion that he stood down from this arduous duty. His sight was very poor. Even producing minutes of a meeting was a massive challenge. Imagine the approach he had to follow. He wrote the first draft in his own handwrit-ing and asked a friend who was unfamiliar with the vocabulary to type it for him. He then sent me a copy to proofread before finding someone else to produce another typed copy and then another friend to circulate it to members. Fortunately, another volunteer was on hand. He was one of my golfing friends. Ronald, who in real life was a professor of veterinary science specialising in large animals, has been a powerful contributor to all aspects of the work of the Group and I relied very much on him for advice and involvement.

We had similar kinds of changes with our treasurer. Joy struggled for well over a year with banks and finance reports. Eventually, we handed over these responsibilities to another volunteer, Colin, who has substantial business and local authority experience. We enjoyed a smooth transfer of responsibilities. The ex-treasurer, Joy, remained a full-time volunteer as a tea lady and as a valuable member of the committee and is truly a joy. Since the transfer of duties with the easier access for Colin to various facilities and amenities, the finances have stabilised. From the beginning, we have avoided asking the members to pay for attending meetings. We placed a box by the tea serving hatch and asked members to contribute to the expenses as they felt able. With the help of some contributions following talks presented by members of the committee to interested groups within the local society, we accumulated around £500 in four years and were pleased to contribute to the Macular Society appeal to support research on macular projects. Also, we make a contribution to the WSBPS who generously share their premises with the Group and help in other ways.

The increase in members has resulted in more, valuable volunteers who responded magnificently to the

Group. Their contributions have been enhanced by their attendance at high-level courses organised at a national level by the Macular Society. Janet, an ex-physics teacher took over the duties of leaflet monitor when the deterioration of Marlene's eyesight made her duties too onerous. Janet then discovered she had a gift for training people to use peripheral vision and is currently helping three members and has given talks to the Group and elsewhere. Christine, from Manchester University, has suffered from Charles Bonnet Syndrome and has given lectures to help on the subject. She trained with the Macular Society on both Charles Bonnet Syndrome and the three-day course encouraged by the Macular Society relating to the use of gadgets as an aid to the management of everyday life. This was a follow-up course to the Macular Society Daily Living Champion course which was created with lottery funds. And then there is Bob. He had a unique experience which persuaded him of the importance of self-awareness of the onset of macular disease and has an almost missionary approach to share this concern. He regularly sets up an information table in places of high footfall in hospitals and is now on the Macular Society list of key speakers. I should also tell you about Doreen, an elderly lady who has been in the Macular Society longer than most and, if pressed, will quietly tell you that she has been a telephone volunteer for the Society for all this time.

Yes, volunteering has many different clothes. Volunteers are a key resource richly encouraged by all support groups who seek to care for others. Late in 2016, our committee decided to have a brainstorming session to think ahead. Christine led the discussions and started by asking each of us to explain why they were comfortable with volunteering and why they had got involved. Everyone mentioned the satisfaction they felt about their involvement. Most had developed some form of eye disease, whilst others had direct experience of loved ones and friends who were struggling or suffering from one form of disease or another. The sense of dedication expressed by my colleagues was very moving. Being involved was worth being involved.

Chapter 7

Walking or Golf?

Long, long ago, certainly before the days when neither one's age or the condition of one's eyes were relevant, my friends and I discussed the unsubstantial question, 'Which would you choose if you had to give up either golf or walking?' My friends chose walking and I chose golf. The prospect of a rational discussion evaded us. This question is irrelevant. Gut feelings were probably dominant. This question is irrelevant for me today because my eyes don't allow me to make a choice except under special circumstances. But, hold on, you have friends and colleagues who still enjoy their golf and have vigorous walks.

I played my first round of golf with a friend in Pittsburg, Pennsylvania when I was thirty-nine years old and I beat him. It was in the depths of winter and the course was covered with a layer of crisp white snow and we were the only people playing. This was the start of a modest career in golf which lasted for many decades and was full of happy times. On my return to England in the early summer, eventually, I got into a good golf club close to home. After a few practice rounds, I managed to achieve a handicap of 16. My skills were rewarded with some success in club competitions which were recognised by getting my name on one – only one – of the honour boards, and my game improved over the years to a handicap of 10. If anyone asks, and they don't, I mention my two holes-in-one, and the match I played in the final of the Captain's Prize in 1977, which I lost on the 16th, to a brilliant 18-year-old who later became a top professional golfer.

One of the joys of golf is to play a round on one of the wonderful courses in the United Kingdom, particularly a course that has hosted one of the famous 'Open' venues and attracted golfers from all over the world: courses like Royal Liverpool, Royal Birkdale, Turnberry and Carnoustie. Part of the fun is to join with others to play on these and numerous other splendid and challenging courses. Early in my golfing career, I joined with three friends and, in true 'Boys Own' style, we formed a unique four strong group which we called 'The Heswall and Cambridge Golfing Society (HCGS). Each member was assigned a specific duty: – secretary, treasurer, fixture secretary and auditor. A detailed report of each four-day yearly outing was deposited in the archives at the local library.

The highlight of all our outings took the Society to the home of golf in St Andrews, Scotland. I still get immense pleasure when I read the report of this trip which I keep with all the other contributions, notes, tee cards, course maps, hotel dockets and short poems or reports written by one of the members, which all hold a fond memory of the fun we had. The Society had to apply in advance for a tee-time on the Old Course at St Andrews, which is the premier course of the seven courses at St Andrews Links. We were thrilled to be drawn to play at 9.30 am on June 16, 1992, and we stood proudly on the first tee when the starter emerged from his wooden hut and shouted, "Play away gentlemen".

Four hours later we had reached the 17th hole, popularly known as the Road Hole and celebrated by many as the toughest hole in the world. The fairway stretches 495 yards. The green is long and narrow and there is a deep cavernous bunker along one side and a road on the other. The archive report shows that all the HCGS team had good drives and that the treasurer hit his second shot into the infamous 'Road' bunker, where it rested up against the steep front wall bordering the green. A small crowd of spectators were amazed to see the treasurer splash his ball out of the bunker to within four feet of the hole. In the enthusiastic applause, one spectator called out, asking for the shot to be played again so that he could get a better photograph!

The HCGS enjoyed over thirty annual outings and played on over a hundred different courses. Each year, the treasurer made a generous subvention from the Society's funds as a contribution to their ladies, who enjoyed their outings to other parts of the United Kingdom. A celebratory dinner of husbands and their wives was held to share memories and agree to repeat the outing next year. Sadly, old age has nibbled at the health of its members and the nearest they get to golf is around a dinner table. The treasure and his lady have succumbed to the throes of the grim reaper and the fixture secretary and his lady have left for another country (Wales).

Even though I have played golf on six continents, with five of them in a single calendar year, and have reminded myself again of how much I have richly enjoyed all aspects of golf, I continue to give preference to walking and I have a very special reason for wishing to mention it in this part of my story – be patient and read on.

I get a walking stimulus every morning of my life as I draw the curtains and look out across the Dee estuary to the Clwydian Hills topped by the 562 metres high peak of Moel Famau. Some call it a mere pimple. It doesn't look as sharp as it did fifty-five years ago when we first arrived in Heswall. I know the path to the tower at the top of Moel Famau like the back of my hand and the hazy view across the water still gives me a good feeling. Our five children have climbed Moel Famau many times and still do. I can't manage to struggle too much more than the halfway bench and I need some friendly support to help me over the rocky parts of the path.

The family was rather slow graduating to the big hills of Snowdonia in Wales and of the Lake District of the north of England. Eventually, I speeded up with the enthusiasm of my close friend, Peter, who was a sailor, not a golfer. One of the problems which slowed my enthusiasm for the hills was in my head. I have a long-term memory of a story from my dad. He told me about his only visit to the Lake District with his friends. They planned to 'do' Striding Edge on the eastern side of Helvellyn which is one of highest peaks in the Lakes. He said, he had been really scared and he hadn't tried it again.

Caution was in our minds the first time we took our family to the Lake District. We called into an information booth in the car park close to the shores of beautiful Lake Coniston and looked up to the towering mountain of Coniston. We sought the advice of one of the Lake District wardens stationed in the booth and we got a very stiff lecture. I think the man in charge was waiting for us! Rather timidly, I asked him to suggest a good path to walk up Coniston. He stood up to his best height and with the authoritarian presence of a schoolmaster, or mountain rescuer, he gave our family all sorts of warnings of the risks involved: sudden changes in visibility, hidden quarry workings, fog and winds. We didn't even set off. Of course, he was right to warn us: essential advice for all hill walkers. It took the enthusiasm and wisdom of Peter to get me out on the Fells to start another great life adventure. Peter led me over many of the trickier climbs in the Lakes including Striding Edge, Jake's Rake, Sharp Edge on Blencathra, the icy screes and steep gullies above Goat's Water near Coniston, and the Terrace on Pillar.

My very first walk with Peter was in the heavy snow around the 11-mile Fairfield Horseshoe from Ambleside. This became an annual 'must walk' for our family. Every year, on my birthday in the middle of August until I reached eighty years of age, up to twenty-five of my accumulated family did the Horseshoe irrespective of weather, and had a wonderful, life-affirming celebration which usually included a fine dinner at a local hostelry paid for by the proud celebrant. Sadly, Peter died after a fight with cancer in 1995. A great man and a dedicated volunteer for many worthy causes.

The story I really want to tell about walking can be traced back to 2008. I was wondering what to do to make life a bit more exciting. Was there a project out there? How about doing the 'Coast to Coast'? This is a big walk which was designed and developed by Alfred Wainwright, the greatest fell walker of our times. It starts at St. Bees in

Cumbria on the edge of the Irish Sea and stretches 196 miles across the north of England to Robin Hood's Bay in Yorkshire, on the North Sea coast near to Whitby. The path opens up the magnificent scenery as it passes three national parks: the Lake District, the Yorkshire Dales, and the North York Moors National Parks. The scenery is magnificent. Some walking enthusiasts take 10 to 12 days to walk the path, only breaking for overnight stops. I decided that my best option would be to take a year and combine shorter walks.

In 2008, as of now, our social activities and holidays were bounded by my wife Pauline's duties as organist at Heswall Methodist Church. She has sole responsibility for playing every Sunday, and often at other times of the week, with no stand-ins or alternatives available. This means that most of our weekends are spent in Heswall and extended holidays are unlikely. At the end of 2008, I had finished my project on the distribution of wildflowers on a piece of heathland adjacent to my garden which has been designated a Site of Scientific Interest, *Wild Flowers on the SSSI,* and so the New Year was wide open – I would do the Coast to Coast.

It didn't take much thought to realise that I would have to do the walk in short sections and would be totally dependent on Pauline ferrying me around the north of England. We devised a plan, which involved taking two or three-day long 'midweek' breaks over the year (2009) staying at comfortable pubs or guest houses; I would walk, and Pauline would explore the countryside by car. An essential part of the plan was that I would need to do daily walks of about 12 miles and that it wasn't necessary to do these in any special order.

The detailed planning was done with the help of Martin Wainwright's book *The Coast to Coast Walk*, with a little help from Alfred Wainwright's book *A Coast to Coast Walk*. The two Wainwrights are not related to each other and the sections of the overall walk were not identical. There is a vast amount of information on the web and Google Earth has been invaluable. BBC TV featured Julia Bradbury in a TV programme called *Wainwright Walks: Coast to Coast*. In preparation, I did some 'health-check' walks mainly on the Wirral Way and on Moel Famau.

My initial feeling about some of the legs was that I would need to be accompanied, for safety's sake, but this didn't happen. However, I did have the pleasure of good company on a few legs and, best of all, Pauline was always there to welcome me and breathe a sigh of relief at the end of each walk.

As part of this project, I produced a 'book', complete with a photographic record, which I hoped would remind me of hundreds of happy and wonderful experiences on my Coast to Coast walk as I moved towards shuffling off this mortal coil.

The Lake District is a wonderful place with spectacular scenery, beautiful lakes and exciting walks and climbs. Wainwright was the type of man who avoided lanes and roads as much as possible. His Coast to Coast has a wealth of tricky ups and downs to challenge even experienced walkers.

I want to tell you about a special experience on one of the legs of my Coast to Coast walk. On 12 April, 2009 (Easter Sunday) we made a speedy escape after Church in

Heswall and arrived 100 miles and two hours later, in glorious sunshine in Ambleside at the edge of Lake Windermere. Dinner at our Ambleside flat was roast breast of duck. There were spectacular views of the Fairfield Horseshoe, Loughrigg, and the Langdale valley. My planned walk on Easter Tuesday was from Stonethwaite in Easedale to Grasmere. Rain was forecast at the higher levels of the walk, but my schedule didn't allow me to choose. The sun broke through at times and I enjoyed a rainbow spanning Stonethwaite Beck as I climbed up Greenup Gill.

I crossed Stonethwaite Beck at Stonethwaite and walked on the eastern side of the Beck, and later Greenup Gill, which has a succession of impressive waterfalls. The massive Eagle Crag dominates this part of the walk. The going got quite tough as I approached Lining Crag. It was wet, windy, nearly in the clouds, and the track was very tricky! It was said that the Lakeland path upgraders had worked here to make the screes less treacherous. Beyond Lining Crag and Greenup Edge (2,000 feet high), the path becomes indistinct and very boggy. There is a long downhill stretch between two lines of long-out-of-use boundary posts before the descent down Far Easedale Gill and Easedale into Grasmere.

It was here that I had a *tortoise and hare* experience that added to the interest of this rather dull walk; probably 'dull' because the weather had closed in. The *hare* was a young and experienced fell walker who moved at a very good pace despite the extremely rugged down-hill walking conditions. The *tortoise* was a group of four men, aged between forty-five and fifty years, who were doing the whole Coast to Coast walk. They were a team in a very special way. One man was almost totally blind. When

I passed the group, one of his colleagues was guiding the blind man step by step over rocks and boulders, the path. A third man walked ahead seeking easier walking conditions for the blind man across the boggy grasslands. The fourth man took off on the alternate peak route over Helm Crag into Grasmere. I supposed that each of the sighted men took it in turns to be the step-by-step guide for the blind man. His colleagues told me that the blind man walked like an express train on the flat and level ground and was difficult to keep up with.

The only other people I saw on the higher stretches of this walk was a team of four teenage girls who I imagined were doing a Duke of Edinburgh assignment, good for them. The whole walk took me over four hours and Pauline was waiting for me in the valley with a lovely home cooked tongue sandwich. We were at Goody Bridge which was the starting point of the next leg to get me to Patterdale on an easier path with splendid views of Striding Edge on Helvellyn and the top of Fairfield. I have a great deal of respect for this blind man and for his friends. My feeling is that many people are willing to help blind people. I will give some other examples, from other circumstances, in a later chapter.

I abandoned long walks and golf over five years ago and although my driving license had over a year to run before the usual three-year renewal period ended, I couldn't help feeling that I was an 'accident waiting to happen' so I decided that this must stop also. Stopping golf was rather more complicated and it would be remiss of me if I didn't conclude with the demise of 'Derek Hull's golfing career'. My handicap was starting to go up and I was losing the joy of watching my shots rise majestically towards the green and settle by the pin. There was also the problem of losing balls that wandered off course into the long grass. For a few months, I had to rely on my playing friends following the ball and tracking it down. But they were ageing at the same rate as me and although they still had a good idea of the direction, they often forgot where it had landed. Young golfers should be aware, this problem will catch up with you eventually. There had to be my last game when I lost four balls in the same round on the ninth hole at Heswall Golf Club. Without a hint of anger but with some regrets, I, rather ceremoniously, said a final goodbye to golf by painstakingly gathering all my golfing clubs, bags, shoes, wet gear, golf balls etc. and taking them to the Oxfam shop. My adventures at the golf course are now limited to the very pleasant Thursday evening dinners at the Club every week, and the gentle company and camaraderie of old, dear friends who even help me by buttering my bread roll.

Chapter 8

Frozen Memories

On November 14, 1966, I was thirty-five years old and employed by the University of Liverpool. We lived in Heswall about 12 miles from the University. There were three sensible ways to travel to the University from our home and I tried them all: by train and bus, by bus and the Mersey river ferry or by car. For speed and convenience, I eventually settled on the latter, but this meant that I had to use the only road tunnel under the River Mersey, pay the tunnel fees and find a place to park the car. The tunnel is called Queensway Tunnel. A second tunnel (Kingsway Tunnel) was being constructed but in 1966 there was little prospect of an early completion to ease congestion. The popularity of living on the Wirral Peninsula was increasing. Queensway Tunnel had two lanes in each direction and was subject to heavy traffic and massive delays. Sometimes my tunnel journeys were a nightmare. There was the prospect of being trapped in one's car inside the tunnel for over thirty minutes. I felt that my time was precious. I decided to write a diary.

I suspect that there are few people who would give such a convoluted excuse for starting a diary. There is also the question – 'Why write a diary?' One approach to answering this last question would be to ask Google to explore how philosophers and thinkers have answered this provocative question. But, this book is supposed to be an autobiography. I will restrict my thoughts to the approach used by Samuel Pepys.

Pepys was a great diary writer. He was born 1633 and lived in London, dying there in 1703. He was distinguished in many ways and an integral part of London life as an MP, Chief Secretary to the Admiralty and Fellow of the Royal Society. His diaries give the impression that he was a constant presence in London. He was a close witness of The Great Fire of London and the Great Plague of London, both of which occurred in the decade of his diary, written between 1660 to 1669. He was also a close observer of the lives of his family, friends and professional colleagues. Pepys had lots of things to write about!

On Monday 14 November 1966, following another long delay in the tunnel, I bought a Collins Ideal Case Bound 578 Feint 160-page Notebook. These notebooks are still available today but now have 192 pages. I started to write my Tunnel Diary, and in the last fifty years, I have filled thirty-six of these notebooks. I estimate that they contain about 1,750,000 words. My last entry was on Thursday 10th November 2016. This entry tells me that on the previous day Donald Trump had become President-elect and that the Hull family, consisting of mum and dad and five grown-up children, had gathered that day for a discussion about the prospects of the 85-year-old founders of the dynasty, downsizing from their home of twenty-five years. The last line of the last page says, "My eyes are very sore, and I can't keep my writing on the lines".

As with Pepys, my diaries were personal. I just wrote what was on my mind without any special agenda. This could be about our family stories, discussions about research and careers, a summary of the events of the day, my views about policy and people, local and world trage-dies, sporting successes and failures, my golf results, health and any amount of tittle-tattle. In summary, I recorded anything that was on my mind at the time of writing. I also used my diaries to sort my mind out and set my priorities. Pepys ensured that his diary was confidential by writing in his own brand of shorthand. Over the years scholars have transcribed his writings and have published collections of his diaries.

I am privileged to have known Robert Lathom, one of the two principal editors of a complete, eleven-volume edition of a transcription of the diaries which include com-prehensive notes and an index. The original diaries are held in the Pepys Library of Magdalene College, Cambridge. For a few years, I was a Professorial Fellow of Magdalene where Robert Lathom, also a Fellow and Pepys Librarian, was completing the final stages of the transcription. Pepys bequeathed his library of three thousand books to the College and the Library with special conditions about the way the books were displayed and maintained. The Library is housed in the Pepys Building at one end of Second Court. For a time, I had rooms on the third floor of this build-ing just above the famous library.

I have often wondered why Pepys stopped writing his diary after nearly ten years. He was only thirty-six years old at the time. In part of his diary, he refers to having sore eyes owing to the strain of so much writing, and I am well aware that detailed microscopy and projects associated with complex graphical work seem to be the cause of my own eye discomfort although I have yet to find a doctor who supports this view. In the Preface to the Lathom Edition, there is a reference to a suggestion that Pepys abandoned the diary in 1669 because of an unfounded fear that he was going blind. His eyesight began to trouble him, and he feared that writing in dim light was damaging his eyes. He did imply in his last entries that he might have others write his diary for him but doing so would result in a loss of privacy and it seems that he never went through with those plans. In the end, Pepys's fears were unjustified, and he lived another thirty-four years without going blind, but he never took to writing his diary again. The diary says that on his last day he was very busy. He spent a lot of time review-ing progress on the construction of his new coach, visiting some colleagues in the Royal Society – Oldenburgh and Wren, and closes with one much said expression, "and so to bed – God give a blessing to it".

Over the years, I have enjoyed writing my diary and the prospect of having to stop because of loss of sight has con-cerned me for a long time. The expression 'frozen memories' seems appropriate. I started to think about how I could keep some accessible records. Indeed, a way of making notes that highlight key events which were in a form that could be read. I opted for an audio approach. To explain this, I must tell you about the way I use my computer. I have had an Apple iMac computer for many years and have made a great deal of use of it as a sighted person for extensive writing and quite a lot of graphics. When I started to lose sight I tried, with some success, to learn to touch-type. Since those early days, the writers of computers programs have produced many modifications to facilitate access to computers for dis-abled people, particularly for those with sight problems. On

Apple computers, these aids are shown under the heading 'accessibility'. The simplest aid is called zoom. It produces, at the touch of a key, a controlled magnification of the screen so that, for example, any text on the screen is enlarged for easier reading. With Voiceover on, the software in the computer transforms text on the screen so that it is spoken by the computer. Finally, there is an accessibility package which transforms sound spoken into a microphone built into the computer which allows speech to be recognised and transformed into text on the screen. These and many other facilities must be learnt before they can be used effectively. The other part of my computer facilities is an Apple iPad which has all the accessibility functions as the iMac. These two computers can be synced by wi-fi so that the information of one is available on the other.

Thus, to write a sentence as in an email, note or paragraph one can dictate the sentence using Siri on the iPad which is displayed as text and then switch on Voiceover and listen to it being read or alternatively print it via iMac. There are many variants to this approach. There is a need for the computer to have a good voice recognition system and I am hoping that this will be achieved in future updates of computer software.

Using this approach, when I still had enough sight to read my hand-written diary, I dictated brief notes to my iPad from the diary and created an abbreviated, dated index to my diaries. This could then be read using Voiceover or used to produce a printed hard copy to be read when a cheap video reader is available on the market. Using the computer search facility all the topics in the abbreviated list can be accessed directly. This makes searching a long hand-written diary possible.

This approach can be used for writing longer texts such as a book but in my experience, it is not quite so simple. One of the main difficulties is that writing a book involves constant checking and rewriting. Producing a smoothly worded text is very difficult with dictation. Making alterations is tedious and time-consuming, so with regret, I have had to steer clear of this method for the writing of this book.

The title of this chapter, Frozen Memories, maybe a clue as to what I had in mind when I started writing my diaries. A diary, no matter who it is written by, is a sort of reminder or insurance against loss of memory or memories. I certainly have difficulty in remembering all sorts of things. Sometimes things are very clear for a long time and others disappear almost immediately. I have great difficulty, for example, remembering a telephone number even walking between two rooms, but the condition is more serious than that. What am I doing? I am writing a diary, thinking in terms of making sure that important things in life are recorded. When I think about how the diary has been used in the last fifty years, it is clear, that it has not been used very much, though I would frequently read a passage or two to reflect on or refresh a memory or a thought for my own pleasure. Within the context of family members, there have been many occasions when the knowledge contained within the diary has been valuable. At times, when family arguments over the details and dates of holidays and all sorts of other events require the certainty of the written word rather than relying on the extraordinary memory of Pauline, it is quite satisfying.

There was an email from Apple recently announcing a new App capable of reading handwritten script and, in the email, there were links to YouTube showing how it is possible to read simple messages such as greetings on Christmas cards with the App. This is not likely to be a universal solution because of the wide range of handwriting styles and quality, but it does offer a hope that some opportunity to read handwriting for partially sighted people is being developed and it is certainly something to be explored.

Now, of course, all the writing in my diary until very recently is handwritten script and, as far as I know, I have no shorthand code that would raise the chance of inadvertently revealing secrets, if it were broken. They can be read by anyone who can read clear, very regular handwriting. You are all welcome. I suspect that this general topic has been of concern for many families when considering what we keep, to remind us of our past parents and families. I very much hope that my diary will be useful in the future, even if not at the same level as those of Samuel Pepys, Captain Robert Scott or Anne Frank, so please don't ask me what I would like to be done with my diaries when my story ends or when there are no more stories to be told. I cannot even think that they deserve to be thrown away, although I recognise the experiences may not contribute to the history books of the last three hundred years in so many ways. I also know that my wife, Pauline, would have loved to have had sight of family diaries from two or three hundred years ago when she was compiling the family trees of the Hulls, Hayes, Scotts and Carrington's of Lancashire and Yorkshire. Perhaps, they would have filled in the ever-present gaps in the history of our families and enlightened us with an insight into the story of their times.

So, sorry folks, perhaps I do wish that my diaries, full of wisdom as they are, should be preserved for posterity.

Chapter 9

Loneliness

I can't remember from my earlier years a time when there was as much talk about the social problems of loneliness as there is in present times. Without having any firm evidence, I suppose that social scientists would agree and attribute the difference to changes in the structure of communities and related topics. I shudder at the potential for loneliness in the new care home at the top of our road which has accommodation for fifty-five single units. Yes, they have lots of mod cons and residents can have their toenails cut and their hair done on request. They also have communal eating and lounges but, well, loneliness?

The potential for isolation and a sense of being neglected must get more acute with ageing accompanied by illness, loss of loved ones and the inability to cope with the trauma of deterioration in mental health. Some health problems such as deafness and loss of sight can be particularly distressing. There was a reminder of these difficulties in a BBC Sunday morning appeal on behalf of The Macular Society. The speaker was the well-known cricket commentator Henry Blofeld, who has glaucoma and has now retired from his cricket job. Similarly, the sense of isolation and loneliness experienced by some blind people is the main feature of the 2017 Christmas Appeal by the Macular Society.

There are about thirty thousand people living in our small town of Heswall on the banks of the Dee Estuary, a few miles from Liverpool, Birkenhead and Chester. In a recent survey, published in the national press, Heswall was described as the third happiest place in Britain. I have no idea how this was determined, but if I had to guess, I would suggest that one of the key factors is the number and effectiveness of networking opportunities which encourages people to talk to each other. There are six different denominations of the church, a wide range of sporting activities including golf, tennis, squash, walking groups, cycling etc. The urge to shop is catered for by five supermarkets, and for those who want to stretch their minds and social activities, there is any number of clubs and pubs. To mention a few: Soroptimists, Rotary, WI, Probus, U3A, Theatre clubs, etc.

When my golfing days were drawing to an end, but before I had to stop playing because of AMD, I became aware, chatting to some men who were showing signs of advancing years, of a club in town called Probus. It had some attractions to me and sounded very friendly and welcoming. The name Probus is an abbreviation of the words Professional and Business, however, membership is not restricted to these two groups. It seeks to embrace anyone who held a position of responsibility during their professional life, providing an opportunity for retired (or semi-retired) professionals to attend regular meetings with like-minded people who appreciate similar interests and social standing. It has been so successful in Heswall that a few decades ago the club, originally called Heswall Probus, had so many members that it split into two separate clubs – Heswall Probus and Gayton Probus. Nowadays each club has about one hundred members. So many men wanted to join Gayton that I was put on a waiting list for new members. When my time came, I was welcomed most warmly after a very brief discussion with the chairman. Probus was set up to provide a support network for retired professionals, so the minimum age for its members is about sixty-five years. Now the average age of its members is just over ninety years old with the occasional member being over 100 years of age. A 90th birthday is celebrated with the gift of a bottle of whisky. Before I reached the age of seventy-two, I rather joked about this group of men who seemed to have given up on life, but I eventually started to envy them as they talked to each other.

Our members are from all walks of life: mariners, doctors, electrical and mechanical engineers, company directors, professors, bank managers, salesmen etc. All have stories to tell but there isn't much talk about the jobs they left behind.

We meet at the Village Hall every Tuesday morning throughout the year. A super team of volunteers arrive early to put out the three bridge tables, a table tennis table and two rows of trestle tables surrounded by chairs, then they put the kettle on ready for morning coffee. When I first joined I enjoyed a game of table tennis, but after a few years, I noticed that the ball disappeared part way along its flight and I realised that the pattern of disappearances coincided with the blind regions shown up by the field of vision monitor at the opticians. Eventually, I had to retire and join the talking classes. Some of my partially sighted colleagues in Probus have managed to graduate to the bridge tables.

The talkers are an interesting lot and usually belong to the senior members' group. There are quite a lot of members who, mainly for health reasons, are unable to attend regularly. They are given the status of permanent apologisers but are kept in touch with the group. Meanwhile, the talkers attempt to solve the problems of the government, the opposition and the world. They regularly relapse into discussions about health. One enlightened member suggested that perhaps we should divide into smaller tables each dedicated to a specific health condition such as hips and knees, dementia, bladder problems, hearts, etc. There would be a lot on the eye table. All would agree with Winston Churchill's observation after a stroke that "Growing old is not for the faint-hearted". At the end of the morning, the fit members put the table and chairs away.

The life of Probus continues in many ways. There is a monthly lunch with a speaker and special parties for our ladies. Our social secretary arranges cultural and industrial visits. There are quiz competitions, bowling and snooker matches against other local Probus clubs. A committee meets at regular intervals and the monthly newsletter keeps everyone in touch. Members willingly drive others to events including funerals of members ... and we don't shout at each other. Mutual goodwill between members abounds and one of our members has special responsibilities in keeping a watchful eye on members who are in failing health.

Most of the organisations listed above, from churches to theatre groups, have open doors for new members and offer many opportunities for social interactions and the chance to meet new people. But I know from my contacts that not all people are joiners and talkers. Not all people have the time and opportunity to escape from difficult circumstances. Some are trapped in mental and physical health difficulties and struggle with a deep sense of loneliness and depression. Many of these feelings are aggravated by personal circumstances and sight loss. The immense value of social interactions cannot be underestimated, and I am lucky enough to enjoy the continued sociability of the Heswall Golf Club, Probus, The Macular Society group and the Methodist Church and the companionship they offer. Often the friendships overlap more than one of these establishments, and the camaraderie is richer for it. With some friends, we have, for many years, been going to a series of concerts at the Liverpool Philharmonic Hall. I have been the annual organiser and ticket buyer. This year the task of purchasing the tickets by a telephone call with the booking office was more of a challenge – particularly settling the account with my credit card on the telephone. I couldn't find my credit card or, when I finally did find it, read the credit card numbers to complete the transaction. The booking clerk, guessing that my sight was very bad, asked me if I had sight problems and if so, was I aware of the scheme which provided a free ticket for an accompanying carer to attend the concerts. Yes, please! And, apparently, similar schemes are available elsewhere. I had no idea! Maybe I will get to keep my job as chief ticket booker for our group of friends for a while longer, and we can continue to enjoy the shared company of a classical concert if only I can find my credit card!

At the beginning of this book, I opined that I had enjoyed a full and satisfying life. The early onset of eye disease leading to AMD has not affected this view, although the progress of the disease is not predictable, and I am still enjoying a positive life. However, it doesn't take much imagination to create or recognise the dark side in relation to loneliness and isolation, and I am not oblivious to the prospect that the developing situations could well be an issue for me in the future. I must think in these terms since I have witnessed a lot of changes in my sight and it seems likely that it will continue to deteriorate further making problem-solving more difficult. It is worth reflecting on how one copes with it in this increasingly technological world we live in. I can recognise signs of frustration as I try to maintain some of my administrative home duties. In the past, I have relied heavily on my computer to keep a check on my current account at my bank so that with the press of two buttons on the computer a full bank statement could be viewed within seconds. Nowadays, I must seek the help of my wife to telephone the bank after searching for all sorts of codes, numbers and passwords to establish that I am who I say I am and that she is a thoroughly reliable person to handle my affairs. It is trivial, but massively frustrating. Alternatively, I can wait for one of my daughters to make a 100-mile round trip and navigate my computer with impressive, but nevertheless infuriating ease.

Ever since the eye disease started, I have recognised the need to find ways, as best I can, to overcome problems and ease difficulties. The good news is that there are many people and organisations willing and able to help – but one has to make the effort to seek that help. The staff in the hospital ophthalmology department directed me to the Wirral Society for Blind and Partially Sighted (WSBPS) which offers a range of aid and facilities for blind people of all ages. The Royal National Institute for the Blind (RNIB) in Liverpool has an even wider range of aids and facilities. One of the gadgets I have found most useful is the Liquid Level Detector – a nifty gadget which attaches to the side of a cup. It can then detect when the liquid being poured into the cup has almost reached the full level and emits a beeping noise to warn you to stop pouring. It can even be adjusted to allow variation in the amount of milk taken in one's tea! Another would be the talking telephone which will speak to you as you type the name or number of the recipient of your call and aims to simplify the use of this vital communication tool. Sadly, for me, it was not quite so simple to master, though I am sure that someone who had been previously familiar with using a mobile phone and texting prior to losing sight would be at a significant advantage and benefit hugely from this gadget. Next door to the RNIB in Liverpool is Henshaw's who offer many training courses and social arrangements for the blind. Closer to home in Heswall we have Helplink who offer a taxi service and many opportunities for social contacts, and Age Concern who are active in so many ways to support the aged. Let me give you an example. After living for eighty-six years, my eyes refused to let me cut my toenails (and my wife never stopped complaining about the holes in my socks), so on one Tuesday morning, I asked a group of talkers at our Probus group where I could find a chiropodist. Quick as a flash I was directed to a local Age Concern Care Home which is visited by a freelance chiropodist on a weekly basis. Great!

On the topic of outside help, I would like to mention the help I have received from the local services of the Visual Impairment Team. Once I was officially designated severely partially sighted I was contacted by the team and they have been invaluable in assessing and facilitating some of the practical needs concomitant with partial sight. One such aid is my white walking stick. The obvious practicality of any stick, as most fell walkers will attest to, is as an aid to walking particularly on uneven ground. As a keen walker,

I have used my fell-walkers stick to ease the strain on weary knees on the long final descents back to the valley from the hilltops. My white stick offers both support and guidance, as it is usually respected by those who can see. Most people are very willing to help the blind – from filling in forms in the bank, to helping to choose a wine in the vast rows of shelves in the supermarket, to crossing busy roads. Heswall has a particularly busy road junction with four sets of automated traffic light signals. At one corner is Eye & Eye and at another Lloyds Bank. One presses a button on the signal box on the traffic lights and waits for the ringing bell or a helping hand to guide you across. As I stand to wait, I am often reminded of Mary Dow Brine's poem, *Somebody's Mother*, which even though it was written over a hundred years ago, captures the sense of vulnerability of the person with the white stick and the response of the passer-by. Thank God for those who pause to ask if they can help.

As I draw to the end of this chapter, I question whether I have achieved what I set out to write and express. Perhaps in the words of John Steinbeck, I am, "In utter loneliness as the writer tries to explain the inexplicable". Or perhaps, it seems so inadequate because of the difficulty of expressing deep emotions about oneself and all the people you get involved with through facing the challenge of loss of sight. In our modern world we think there should be no loneliness, and certainly, we all seek to avoid the pain of being alone. It is through a community that we find the answer for as Tennessee Williams so aptly said,

"When so many are lonely as seem to be lonely, it would be inexcusably selfish to be lonely alone."

Somebody's Mother

The woman was old and ragged and gray
And bent with the chill of the Winter's day.
The street was wet with a recent snow
And the woman's feet were aged and slow.

She stood at the crossing and waited long,
Alone, uncared for, amid the throng
Of human beings who passed her by
Nor heeded the glance of her anxious eye.

Down the street, with laughter and shout,
Glad in the freedom of 'school let out',
Came the boys like a flock of sheep,
Hailing the snow piled white and deep.
Past the woman so old and gray
Hastened the children on their way.

None offered a helping hand to her -
So meek, so timid, afraid to stir
Lest the carriage wheels or the horses' feet
Should crowd her down in the slippery street.

At last came one of the merry troop,
The gayest laddie of all the group;
He paused beside her and whispered low,
"I'll help you cross, if you wish to go."

Her aged hand on his strong young arm
She placed, and so, without hurt or harm,
He guided the trembling feet along,
Proud that his own were firm and strong.
Then back again to his friends he went,
His young heart happy and well content.

"She's somebody's mother, boys, you know,
For all she's aged and poor and slow,
And I hope some fellow will lend a hand
To help my mother, you understand,
If ever she's poor and old and gray,
When her own dear boy is far away."

And 'somebody's mother' bowed low her head
In her home that night, and the prayer she said
Was "God be kind to the noble boy,
Who is somebody's son, and pride and joy!"

Mary Dow Brine (1816–1913)

Chapter 10

Why?

It is good to ask questions and struggle with possible answers. At the beginning of this book, I asked a question, and I want to end with two questions which are rather on the fringes of the main topic, but relevant to living with blindness. I still remember, with some embarrassment, as a raw 18-year-old schoolboy, being interviewed by a professor of education at the University of Liverpool when I was trying to gain admission. After the niceties of the first part of the interview, the professor asked, rather quietly: "What is physics?"

I am hoping that my questions will help me to discuss some topics, not yet covered in the book, which seem to be quite important. The first question is: 'Why have I got Age-related Macular Degeneration (AMD) which means that I am nearly blind?' I hope that this question will take me to the importance of scientific research. The second question is: 'Why me?' and then onto the big challenge of finding a way of living comfortably with being blind, which for some people might be developed to the meaning and purpose of life. Tough questions.

One question usually triggers many more, however, there is a little voice in my head telling me that I haven't sufficient knowledge of the ways in which the body works or the underlying science to explain or understand it. But, hold on Derek; since you were diagnosed in the eye department and told that you had AMD, you have heard numerous lectures and meetings and received piles of guides and documents about AMD, from well-meaning sources backed up by reports in newspapers, radio and TV, that you should be able to recognize reasons for some of the following questions about AMD: Is it related to one's genes and DNA? Is it affected by smoking or drinking? Is it caused by having atrial fibrillation and high blood pressure? Is it affected by physical exercise? For myself, until recently, I didn't think genes had anything to do with AMD, but then my brother was diagnosed with the condition.

In the past five years our local Macular Support Group, which meets every other two months, has had the benefit of hearing many talks about research on some important topics in the University of Liverpool by leading academics. Being effectively a new group, we had many discussions about the most suitable subjects for inclusion in a pro-gramme alongside talks on guide dogs for the blind and diets for the blind. There has been a keen interest in talks about medical subjects even though the talks were quite complicated and often beyond the understanding of our members. I felt that our members appreciated the opportu-nity to hear about advanced research even though they fully recognised that the beneficiaries would probably be a later generation. The Support Group has welcomed two talks by our local senior AMD clinician. There were many questions.

Patients familiar with eye clinics will be aware of the wide range of specialised equipment used to diagnose the many different eye conditions. In my experience, the usual first step is the Snellen alphabet chart followed by the field of vision hemisphere. This progresses to more sophisticated, complex observations with a microscope and photography of the many complex layers at the back of the eye, some of which are no more than a few hundreds of microns thick. Where necessary, the clinician may further acquire information using powerful scanning techniques such as magnetic resonance imaging (MRI) and computed tomography (CT scans). I recall being examined by MRI to determine the state of the very fine blood vessels at the back of my eye behind the retina, and by CT scanning to check for signs which might be a haemorrhage associated with a stroke or a Charles Bonnet event.

These types of equipment are used for research into the structure and condition of the eye by scientists in university and other laboratories and highlights that research into eye problems is very expensive. There are many other expensive facilities relating to the vast amount of scientific activity which are an integral part of the whole. I suppose, though I can't, as a layman in these matters, give chapter and verse to expand this statement, that the foundation for diagnostic methods used in determining the eye problems experienced by a patient is based on many decades of detailed scientific studies. Some of these studies will have been related to specific eye conditions identified by clinicians but there will have been contributions from many branches of science. This makes an adequate answer to the 'Why?' question difficult. It does emphasise the importance of providing high-quality science education in our schools.

As a material scientist and engineer, who has spent a lifetime studying the way in which the internal microstructure affects the properties of materials and the ways in which it can be modified to achieve specific properties and performance, I have had many opportunities to demonstrate the value of collaboration between different scientific disciplines. I was involved with the government supported research and engineering committees responsible for the allocation of substantial research grants and resources for a variety of subjects across science, engineering and medicine. On a much smaller scale, I supervised PhD students and research assistants whose work was associated with medical problems which interfaced with science and engineering. This experience was valuable and gave me a strong insight into the importance of collaboration and interdisciplinary projects. As demonstrated by the developments in fields such as dental and ophthalmic surgery, vascular and microsurgery, and heart and brain surgery, to name just a few, the rewards for collaboration can be enormous. Many projects start on a small scale and grow into multimillion pound ventures.

My wife has recently had cataract surgery in both eyes. Millions of people from all over the world have had cataract operations which are now regarded as one of the most successful surgical procedures. The story of the origin of this operation is well worth telling.

Harold Ridley, later Sir Harold, was trained as a medical doctor and later became an ophthalmic surgeon. In World War II, he served in the Royal Air Force and treated eye injuries. One of his patients sustained a splinter in his eye from a damaged cockpit of his aeroplane. The cockpit window was made of Perspex, and Harold Ridley noted that the splinter, although a foreign body, didn't cause any inflammatory reaction in the pilot's eye. Perspex is the trade name for a transparent polymethyl methacrylate (PMMA) which can occur in a very wide range of forms. It is a thermoplastic and is readily transformed into different shapes by heating and moulding. Ridley and his colleagues realized that there was the possibility of using PMMA, suitably shaped, as a replacement lens for patients with cataracts. Ridley performed his first surgery in 1949 at St. Thomas' Hospital, London. Many years of detailed research were required to develop this brilliant first step into a product that is now produced in millions at an inexpensive price. The Inter Ocular Lens was born, and many improvements followed with the development of a new polymer which remains transparent in the eye. This polymer is readily shaped to match the eye and is suitably flexible to be folded to allow the lens to be inserted through a small hole in the front of the eye.

So, we can see that the cataract procedure is a good example of the way an idea can start from small beginnings and develop into a life-changing surgery accessible to thousands of patients a year.

I am reminded of the mornings when our children left home for school on exam days and they heard the dulcet tones of their dad telling them to read the questions. It is the best advice I could give them. Under my breath I might have added; 'And be sure to answer the questions on the exam paper and do not create in your head another question that you could answer'. I sense that this advice is relevant to my response to the first question in this chapter. 'Why have I got Age-related Macular Degeneration (AMD)?" Although I can't answer the main question, I have drawn the conclusion that this discussion about research highlights the following:

1. A lot of medical resources are committed to treating AMD.
2. A lot of expensive medical equipment is available in NHS hospitals for diagnostics and care.
3. Many eye problems require further research.
4. There is evidence from many branches of medicine of the importance of a multidisciplinary approach.
5. The key decisions in identifying research projects must rest with the medical expertise.

I am inclined to put all these thoughts against the few things I know about the Macular Society appeal for funds to support research, and in passing, I must admit that my knowledge is limited to what I have read in the Macular Society literature. By initiating a research appeal a few years ago, the Macular Society has emphasized the importance of research for a solution in the treatment and prevention of eye problems. They have been very successful with over £4.5 million being raised in the past five years with more support from the government and the public. These funds are valuable to researchers and they can be used very effectively to initiate new research ventures and help support research staff, particularly in universities. I think there is a need for a fuller understanding of the importance of this funding. In the context of the support for science, £4.5 million is trivial but it can have a massive contribution which may not be fully understood. This is amply demonstrated by the cataract story. In the early stages the costs would be low, whereas once progressing into the areas of development and manufacture, the costs rise dramatically. I learnt this lesson in my early days in university research when I was trying to build up my research group. Rather out of the blue, I was approached by a manager from a research-dedicated chemical company who was keen to encourage my research team to develop ideas in a particular field. He arranged for my university research account to be gifted £3,000 (a lot of money in today's terms) which was to be spent entirely at my discretion. In a sense, I spent this money many times because I primarily used it to initiate small projects, which went on to attract large funds from elsewhere. I was then able to repay the original £3,000 into the university research fund from new free monies. This allowed me subsequently to initiate other new projects and so the process repeated. I used to call this my 'slush fund' and from that original gift stemmed many interesting and productive research programmes which might otherwise not have got off the ground.

There will always be the 'Why?' question and progress towards an answer will be important for diagnosis and for the development of effective treatments and medicines. In respect to AMD, the answer remains incomplete and we must wait awhile for the science to progress.

And so, to my second question, 'Why me?' The answer to the first part of 'Why me?' must surely be highly subjective and be buried in the whole life package of the individual. I have tried to map out my answer, but it is a life story and another book. Some of the answers to the second part may be found in the chapters of this book.

I would start with the affirmation that I am a scientist. I am also comfortable, having had a lifelong involvement with the life of the Christian church, with the view that the Bible is a faithful description of man's experience of God since time began, and relevant to many religious persuasions. So, one can speak of faith in God which is available for all, if it helps. Faith is recognition and acceptance. It is intimate to the individual and provides a basis for coping and rejoicing in the life we have. So, a Christian prays, and a scientist accepts. Unless I can manage this dilemma, there is a danger of missing the wonder which is life and my wish that all humankind receives a blessing.

The premise in science is that things are not absolute; instead, they exist in relation to everything else and can be qualified or diminished by interaction with other factors. Darwin, in the mid-nineteenth century, proposed the concept of an adaption of living species to the environment driven by natural selection with two arguments: firstly, that life evolves from common ancestors and secondly, that life evolves by means of natural selection and adaptation. It has become increasingly apparent that whilst microevolution – small changes over a short-term – may play by these rules, macroevolution is governed far more chaotically with the dynamics of an interaction between the actual organism (hundreds of thousands of genes) and all its traits or observable characteristics (phenotypes) and its environment. When considered in depth, this approach fits comfortably with the scientific understanding of the world and the fragility of life as influenced by chance.

When trying to understand the 'Why me?' question, one inevitably tries to find a reason. One might liken it to a foundation or an anchor from which a sense of security or faith can evolve. A human comfort blanket; predictable and meaningful. When the cause of the question is related to the human body, then the hope is that an answer can be found with an understandable logic. Did I spend too many hours looking down a microscope? Did poor lighting conditions cause Samuel Pepys's sight to diminish? Is it in my genes? To leave the explanation to the brief word of 'chance', could leave one feeling unsatisfied. Chance is an uncomfortable thing. And yet, it became the fundamental basis for Darwin's later work in which he used randomness as a way to explain natural phenomena. For example, whilst there is variation in the length of a giraffes' neck, it is the length that allows him to reach the leaves high on a tree. The longer the neck, the higher the probability of survival. Why do some giraffes have longer necks than others? Darwin put this down to chance, that the cause of the variable is unknown. Around the same period, a French mathematician and physicist, Jules Henri Poincarè stated that when, "A small cause which escapes our notice determines a considerable effect that we cannot fail to see, then we say the effect is due to chance."

It would seem, that there is no simple reason to be found and that maybe the answer to the question 'Why me?' can only go as far as to say that nature will not let herself be predictable. Science can take us a long way along the road of explanation, but even with the benefit of hindsight, we can no more predict the future than look back and find the answer to 'Why me?' There are too many variables. The way we live our lives, and the results and consequences of our choices, can be linked but not as a fixed sequence.

The Butterfly Effect or the Chaos Theory shows that the things that change the world are the tiny things, so tiny they go unnoticed. In the 1950s, Edward Lorenz, a meteorologist and mathematician, was looking for a way to accurately predict the weather. He was using a computer to analyze reams of inputted data in an attempt to produce a weather model that could be applied worldwide. However, he noted that when the starting conditions of the parameters such as wind speed, temperature etc. were altered by a tiny amount, the outcome amplified and the whole prediction changed completely. Lorenz used the Butterfly Effect as a symbolic representation of his findings when he explained in his lectures that a butterfly fluttering from flower to flower in Mexico, has the potential to create tiny changes which, while not creating a typhoon in China, could alter its path. A flapping butterfly wing represents the minuscule changes in atmospheric pressure, and these changes compound as a model progresses. In predicting the weather, the butterfly is the unknown quantity that tips the system, and this concept is the sole reason why weather forecasts begin to be flawed a day or two into the future. The butterfly flapped its wing by chance, and the essence of chaos theory is that a scientist cannot calculate the odds of that occurring. Maybe now we should have more sympathy for Michael Fish who failed to tell the nation that the hurricane of 1987 was approaching.

My own experience of the butterfly effect can be expressed in a real story of a colleague in my hometown. He was driving to work on a very windy day, through a small coppice, when a tree was blown down and fell across the road, hitting my colleague's car and killing him. Such is the fragility of all things that if he had had one more spoonful of cornflakes for breakfast he would or might still be alive today.

However, one thing is certain, that science should continue looking for the butterflies. The explosion in information technology of recent years shows us how small changes can transform the way people live their lives, and while fads come and go, persistent small changes are the most effective way to produce the metaphorical typhoon.

Have I found an answer to 'Why me?' Did I answer the question I was given? In all probability, and to my scientific mind, then yes. Do I have a reason or a point of blame for my failing eyesight? No, the butterfly remains elusive. Genomics tells us that it is statistically unlikely that you inherited any genetic material from your ancestors beyond the ninth generation, but this becomes immaterial as we have no evidence to support a genetic link other than my brother who also suffers from AMD, and the variables are vast. Recent discoveries in relatively new sciences such as Epigenetics, the study of anything which alters gene activity or expression without changing DNA, tells us that genes need instructions: what to do, where and when to do it. These instructions come from gene tags which are triggered by lifestyle and environmental factors. They can be switched on and switched off causing an epigenetic drift, which can come from generations before us and will continue for generations after us. But, I will settle for randomness. Life is always unique, changing and unpredictable, and whatever skills, talents, faults, flaws, or character traits you have, whatever self you were born with, is a product of random variation. My grandchildren might describe it in the words of Forrest Gump: "Life is a box of chocolates, and you never know what you are going to get!"

I offer these thoughts as I struggle with how to accept that I am facing total blindness and try to find a way of avoiding suffering. Despite my present life being restricted as it is by severe partial sight, which has a massive effect on some aspects of the quality of my life, I consider myself fortunate and, as I observed in Chapter 1, life doesn't owe me anything. I hope that I can apply myself to taking full advantage of all the care and support I am surrounded by, in the hope that I can minimize my suffering, and in turn, help minimize the suffering of others similarly afflicted.

There is plenty of evidence in this book for the negative effect of losing sight, and I hear stories of people who struggle to keep cheerful when they are deprived of so many familiar pleasures, from watching TV to shopping at Tesco. I will have the struggle to find things to do particularly when I finish writing this book. Peace and quiet are key targets but this is a tough one to quantify to the reader. There is another side to the author of this book; he is not only a serious scientist but someone who sees the poetry in life, not just the literal. When I go into quiet modes I think about calm and tranquillity; I don't think about electron microscopes, even though they dominated my life at times. This is my peace and quiet, this is my comfort. A time when one doesn't set off with the aim to think, and yet you have a vacuum, and thoughts float in as images pass you by, thoughts which aren't invented or invited, they just arrive. Peace and quiet.

I do get a lot of comforts listening to my print reader to *The Pembrokeshire Odyssey* which I wrote a few years ago when my AMD was showing signs. It is copied at the end of this book (Appendix X). I think I will have a listen now.

Appendix X

The Pembrokeshire Odyssey – September 2014

Introduction

Over the years, we have enjoyed many family holidays in Pembrokeshire in Wales, enjoying the splendid beaches and cliff walks. It is a great place for peace and quiet and for general relaxation. Nowadays, Pauline and I go alone for just a few days. It is wonderful, and our holiday starts as soon as we jump in our VW Golf. We love to drive down through Wales, as every mile of the road is rich in beautiful countryside. After crossing the River Dee at Chester, we pass through the southern end of the Clwyd Hills heading towards Aberystwyth. The route takes us alongside Lake Bala through the foothills of Snowdonia National Park on to Dolgellau with the magnificent Cader Idris framing our view for many a mile. We pass through the historic market town of Machynlleth, before calling in for a coffee at the fine RSPB site Ynys Hir on the Dyfi estuary. Our first real glimpse of the coast is at Aberystwyth and we follow it for a further 80 miles along Cardigan Bay, stopping for lunch on the quayside of Aberaeron, before reaching St Davids at the tip of the Pembrokeshire peninsula. Hopefully, we arrive before 4 pm and after checking into our hotel, we make a dash for Whitesands Bay for our first paddle of the holiday.

My Tunnel Diaries tell me that all my life I've been struggling to 'unscramble' my brain. The short-term treatment or solution is to make a list to clarify the challenges and this reduces them in size.

In September 2014, my brain was completely scrambled, the result of many months of activity and the accumulation of numerous jobs needing completion.

As we drove to St Davids, 'unscrambling' was high on my list of things to think about on our six-day holiday for the year while we pottered around Pembrokeshire. We had chosen a good hotel that would look after us in a quiet and peaceful environment with a minimum of fuss. The weather promised to be very good – sunny and warm – and it was.

For me, unscrambling always starts with identifying and listing the routine, day to day jobs so that there is the time and space to let other thoughts come into my brain. Where does one go when the 'routine' unscrambling list is off the agenda? One stands and stares to allow time and circumstance to have their say – not in any military way but giving the neurons the opportunity to determine the agenda.

So, here goes on a brief Pembrokeshire Odyssey, not an epic Greek poem, more a gentle journey.

We had our banana and crispy bread roll picnic lunch beside a babbling brook in the tiny village of Middle Mill about a mile from Whitchurch, which is close to an abandoned airfield. The babbling brook is the River Solva which winds its way to the sea at Solva. Middle Mill attracts tourists because of the wool mill which spans the tiny river. The mill is reached by a stone bridge over the river. Rising above the village is a narrow road leading to an old church surrounded by gravestones and close by, on the hillside, is a dedicated cemetery still open for the bodies of the dead and the tears of those left behind.

A slight breeze, with the hint of a chilling wind, came down the valley from the north, so Pauline retreated to the car and the *Daily Telegraph* Sudoku, and I wrapped a thick blanket around my shoulders so that I could enjoy sitting in the sunshine as I scribbled on my notepad. Earlier, we had shared in Choral Eucharist at St David's Cathedral with a goodly crowd led by the Dean (Jonathan Lean).

I don't need a cathedral service to introduce me to other mind dimensions, but it helps. The robust preacher used a verse from St Paul's Acts of the Apostles for his text and sermon and told us of the knocking down of whitewashed walls. I didn't really get it all and promised myself that I would look it up later. I did get the sense that there are deeper things to be aware of in the journey of the spirit, or should I say Spirit (whatever that means). I reflected on all the transcendental experiences that cannot be fully grasped making it hard to take them on board in everyday life. They flutter in and out of one's mind like a butterfly moving across the flowers on the bank in the wild part of my garden – never still long enough to really look at them, but real all the same – and when clouds cover the sun they disappear only to reappear when the sun escapes. As I write and relax in this secluded valley, a beautiful red admiral rests on the corner of my garden chair, the first butterfly I have seen all day.

Should I start thinking about dying and death? – no reason for this choice. How about old age? How about a life stripped of self? So many other things fade into the background. At dying and death we leave everything behind, nothing matters, all the pressures that life brings disappear, there is no agenda or forward plan or Quo Vadis or lonely list. As we move into this inevitable state, should we think in terms of a gradual approach to death? What does that mean? Is 'be still my soul' part of the mission statement? Well, that approach hasn't got me very far!

And now, as a wren, or perhaps it was a robin, twitters backwards and forwards across the babbling brook, I realise that I am finding all this broad-brush philosophizing too difficult to grasp. Should I attempt to select some specific issues to bring something into a sharper focus for me, Derek, at eighty-three years? *Ulysses** insists that, despite failing abilities, I should keep the flag flying, but this is not a sufficient or adequate response. Our House Group is preparing a service on the theme, 'What a wonderful world', but this is not adequate either. Much of my peace in the last few years, admittedly spasmodically, has come from poetry and writing storybooks I call cameos. There is often a poem or cameo struggling to find time in a ridiculously busy life. The last cameo I would have liked to explore was about Stoner, John Williams story about a poor American academic whose paths through life were far from smooth, but time, precious time, was elusive and my sight was struggling.

There is a sense that having completed a significant unscrambling of the 'routine' there should be space for thinking about the 'inner life' and my mind drifts to thoughts of my study. Space is far too cluttered, busy, too many agendas, too much useless technology – and then I look up and see a weary old man supported by his son. They are walking slowly along the banks of the stream pausing for a while beside a small tree at the water's edge. As they approach me they stop to talk. The old man lives in London but regularly visits his son in Pembrokeshire. A few years ago, he sought permission to plant a willow tree, which he visits regularly, to remember his departed wife. And then another man joins me to ask if I am painting and we find ourselves talking about writing a diary. I am not making much progress on mind unscrambling – or perhaps I am.

The following day it is warm and sunny with glorious blue skies. As creatures of habit we are in the car park at Saint Govan's Head, the views and coastal path are more than an adequate reward for the long drive. After a walk along the cliff tops and another banana picnic, I am sitting on the cliff tops above the steps down to Saint Govan's chapel. The sea views are quite spectacular. Peace is all around even with some walkers chatting excitedly – they are Welsh. My mind goes back to the previous day when I walked from the coastal path to the Warpool Court Hotel in the early evening. I could hear the cathedral bells calling worshippers to Choral Evensong. More peace, but it isn't helping me focus on mind unscrambling. Just try!!

There is a challenge. Do I want to 'accept' my eighty-three years with a weakened body, fewer mental facilities, loss of fuel in the tank, aches and pains, etc.? What is involved in accepting it? Do I have an option? Do I always have to be doing things, striving to be creative, being active for 15 hours every day, filling all available time (actively, creatively, usefully) as if that is God's calling (expressed in theological language), is it okay to waste time (the time we have been given on God's earth)? Is there a counter-argument that we should give more time and space to doing nothing? And how does all this fit in with the inevitable prospect of more weakening and dying? This sort of space could be very creative, but I don't seriously exercise it, although I do spend a lot of time thinking and reflecting. Perhaps the best thing I can do is put it on the agenda for the next meeting!

The sun is still shining on our last day in Pembrokeshire. I am sitting in the gardens of our hotel looking across the fields to St Non's Retreat Centre beside St Non's Chapel and beyond the misty sea. We are off to Whitesands later. An ambulance is screaming on the high road. Someone is ill or injured or killed. Relatives are sorely distressed, an ambulance crew is anxious, life will change, lives will change. It is the moment, in the twinkling of infinite time, there is no return only going forward. What do the Sisters in the Retreat pray about? When I spoke to one of the Sisters as she was closing the building site she wished me good-bye with 'God bless you'. What do the retreaters think and pray about? What do those burdened with senior moments think about? What do my fellow guests at the hotel think about? Why bother thinking at all, and what if we cannot think? Too many questions – no answers.

Why bother thinking? There are no answers. The old sit on the promenade watching people go by. Why bother? Surely, alongside the long list of routine activities identified earlier, there ought to be space to be comfortable in oneself without any 'mission' element, no prizes at the end, as we slip into eternity. And here, under the trees, the leaves of Autumn are falling making their own noisy signatures. They will produce more leaves in the Spring but like me, they will eventually produce their last leaf and join the path to maximum entropy.

So, can *Ulysses** accept that the six-day mind adventure is completed, however inadequately, and sit back and let untroubled time pass by?

Ulysees, by Alfred, Lord Tennyson, 1833

"Happiness is a butterfly, which when pursued,
is always just beyond your grasp,
but which, if you will sit down quietly,
may alight upon you."

Nathaniel Hawthorne

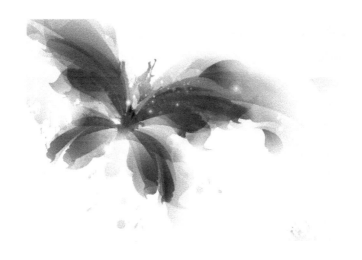

Lightning Source UK Ltd.
Milton Keynes UK
UKHW020713101118
332108UK00005B/160/P